Echography in anesthesiology, intensive care and emergency medicine: A beginner's guide

Springer

Paris
Berlin
Heidelberg
New York
Hong Kong
Londres
Milan
Tokyo

Frédéric Greco

Echography in anesthesiology, intensive care and emergency medicine: A beginner's guide

With the contribution of:
Doctor Jacques Provost, Doctor Alain Boularan, Mr. Roger Pascal

Translated from French by Pauline Lieven

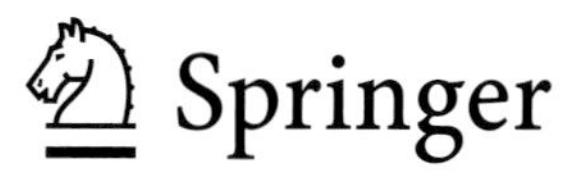

Frédéric Greco
Unité de réanimation du SARC-C
Pôle neurosciences - Tête et cou
Hôpital Gui de Chauliac
80, Avenue Augustin Fliche
34295 Montpellier Cedex 5
f-greco@chu-montpellier.fr

ISBN : 978-2-8178-0015-8 Springer Paris Berlin Heidelberg New York

Printed in France

Springer-Verlag France is member of groupe
Springer Science + Business Media

This book has been translated from the French edition of the book *Échographie en anesthésiologie et en médecine d'urgence*, published by Sauramps Médical in 2008
ISBN : 978-2-84023-556-9

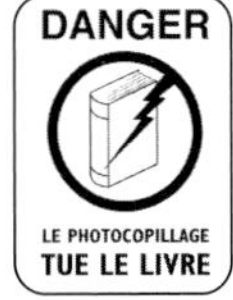

Cover design: Nadia Ouddane
Layout: Graficoul'Eure

To my father
To my mother
To my family
To my friends
To my country

To Our Father

To Doctor Joseph Biban

Contents

Preamble

At the beginning of this century, as I was isolated, on duty in a peripheral hospital, I decided to master the ultrasound tool. This first path was followed by the creation of various trainings. Resulting from approximations, mistakes, and beliefs, this book only pretends to show you what is simple. In these few pages, we have aimed to condense the basic essentials to make your initiation into ultrasound easier.

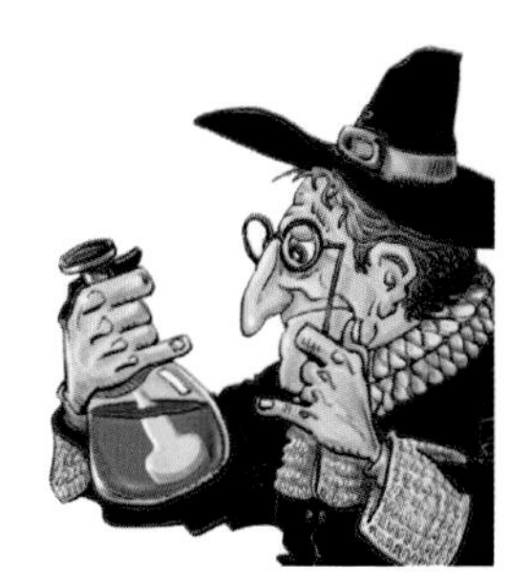

One day, newly transferred into a hospital located on a small island far from any metropolis, I took over from the only anesthesiologist who officiated between the basement and the roof of the hospital. In short, I was alone. Exhausted, my predecessor had been dismissed and warmly taken to the first boat due to leave. With a mischievous smile, he had just had the time to wish me good luck... Odd, isn't it?

Quickly overwhelmed by the job, I begged for mercy and asked for an appointment with the hospital director.
– "Help? Of course, dear doctor, that's absolutely normal."
Surprised by the absence of resistance, I thought with all speed, looking for the trick, and enquired about the practical details.
– "By the end of the week, you will receive help."
With this comforting sentence, I went back to work, full of hope.
As the end of the week was getting closer and closer, I didn't know if I was to be roasted, simmered, or skewered.

Thus, I welcomed the announcement of the arrival of the long-awaited help. Abandoning my syringe, laryngoscope and breathing apparatus, I dashed for the recovery room and joined mister Director with the long-expected help. One incongruous detail however, my reinforcement looked like a car salesman: suit, tie, and pointed shoes.

This is how I found out that the so-awaited human help was actually a material one, an advanced hand-held echograph and, moreover, on a carriage! The Director seemed not to notice my cries and let me fidgeting, congratulating himself he had such a well-equipped operating suite.
The friendly salesman, who seemed a little uncomfortable, quickly regained the upper hand and unveiled the three boxes next to him. **But why three boxes?**
Three boxes because echographs are made of:
- a computer, or button box, with a keyboard, a more or less big screen and a socket;
- probes, transmitters, and receivers with ultrasound systems to be plugged in the button box;
- and a cart to carry the whole apparatus and the very essential printer to keep images of the examination.

In the **first box** was the carriage with supports for probes and gel, two shelves, and two places for a display system and a CD-DVD burner. I couldn't believe my eyes. We were assembling THE all-terrain echograph! But it was not the end of my surprises.

What was hidden in this much smaller **second box?** Where was this echograph? Was it inflatable? Opening the box, I told myself there was a problem because the salesman was handing me a laptop. Nothing to do with an echograph, I thought. What would this material serve for? "But this is the echograph" he told me. *"Take it and weigh it. It is only 4.5 kg. It's a real technology wonder."* Yeah? Right! But, as this technology can neither be on duty rotation nor answer to the beeper, I wasn't out of the woods yet... However, we must admit that, once opened, the computer looked like an echograph with as many buttons as we could wish.

The **third box** contained three probes. **But why were there three?**

- The **first one is a linear probe**. It's a high-frequency probe (5 to 13 MHz) that provides an excellent quality of image. It is used for any superficial examination (4 to 6 cm deep) such as vascular access, regional anesthesia, and study of neck and limb vessels.

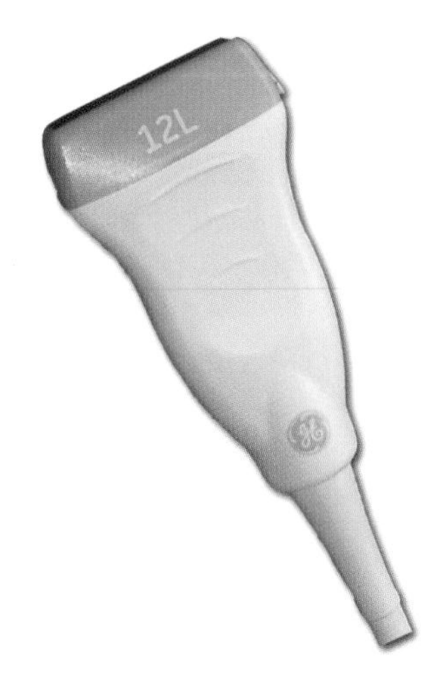

• The **second one, the abdominal probe**, has a rounded form, slightly convex. It uses lower frequency (2 to 5.5 MHz), which offers a good image quality for deeper echographic examinations, that is to say beyond 6 cm and until 20 cm.

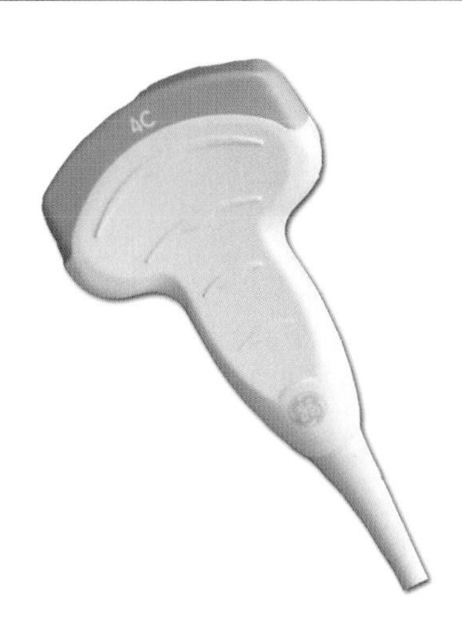

• The **third one is a phased-array probe.** Using low frequency (1.5 to 4 MHz), it is small and square. It gives a triangular image print. Since it is small and provides a good image quality, this probe permits to reach more difficult areas that were impossible to see with the previous probes. It is mainly used in cardiology and makes the way through intercostal spaces easier.

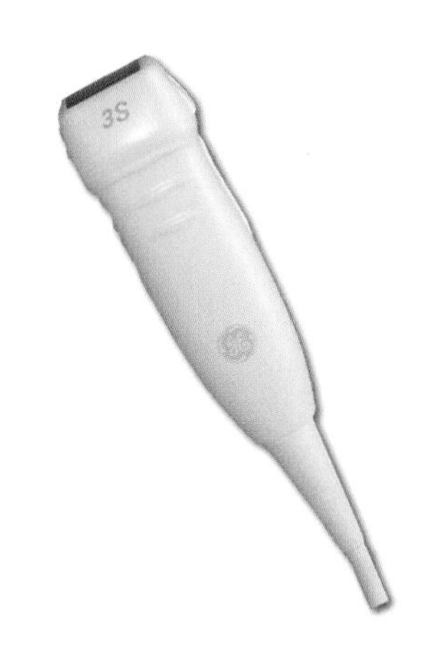

The salesman did his best to break the ice, while seeing we obviously didn't lack it on this island. He struggled to assemble, before my tearful eyes, the technological Lego that was supposed to solve all my problems. Suddenly, with a forced smile, he told me everything was ready. He made a brief presentation during which the different shades of gray followed each other on the display screen. "Anyway, it's very simple!" he told me. And then, brandishing several books with countless pages, not to forget the CD with the digital version, he finished his presentation shouting out "Everything is in the instructions." As he didn't want to miss the last boat, he left me, telling how much he admired my craft.

Distraught, I saw every hope of help fading away and considered the future under bad auspices. And so I neglected the machine and resumed work. All of a sudden, my colleague (a radiologist, by the way) turned up at the operating room and, without any ceremony, embraced me wholeheartedly. Worrying about this very expressive behavior, I feared the worst and, freeing myself, tried to catch the Haloperidol syringe in order to deal with the most urgent matters first. *"My dear friend! What a joy! Oh yes, what a joy! At last my wishes come true because I have an alter ego who will support me."* As I couldn't believe my ears, I asked him to immediately explain himself. *"Yes, my dear friend. With this new apparatus, you will lend me a hand and I will, at last, be able to sleep."*

It was no good my trying to explain to him I had never turned on an echographic machine; he took me under his wing and gave me an article about echography he had written in the past for some friends.

Ultrasounds, a much reflected system

■ Introduction

Although the first publication on the use of ultrasounds to image the human body appeared in 1937, it was only during the sixties that it was first used for medical diagnosis. Since then, the first echograph evolved from expensive, big, immobile machines to compact, mobile machines with all possible features: B-mode, TM, Doppler, 3D...

Besides, the physics principles remained unchanged. In order to obtain as much as possible from using ultrasounds for a medical diagnosis and reduce the risk of errors or artifacts, one must understand the physical and technological bases of ultrasound.

■ Physics bases

Sound is a mechanical wave that is transmitted through longitudinal movements in elastic surroundings. Ultrasound is a sound with a frequency superior to 20,000 hertz (Hz). The ultrasounds used for medical diagnosis have a frequency between 1.5 and 25 megahertz (MHz).

■ Production and propagation of ultrasounds

The ultrasonic beam is produced by a probe (or transducer) that is placed in contact with the skin. We can find a row of piezoelectric crystals within the probe. These crystals have a particular feature: they can change their shape when submitted to an electric flow.

The electrical stimulation that makes the crystal oscillate at its resonance frequency permits to convert the electrical energy into sound energy.

The sound wave spreads through tissues and provokes interactions between the tissues and the sound wave. If the sound goes through a homogeneous tissue, the main interaction is **absorption** of sound wave. The absorbed sound energy is converted into caloric energy. In most cases, this is not hazardous because caloric energy is very weak and quickly vanishes. Nevertheless, we have to take it into account while examining a fetus or an eye. Generally speaking, remember that the output power must be as low as possible all the while giving adequate images. The quantity of absorbed energy is lower in liquid structures than in solid ones.

Most of tissues in the body are not homogeneous; hence, the ultrasonic wave bumps into a **series of interfaces** (limit between two different surroundings). They can be macroscopic (vessel wall) or microscopic (inner structure of the renal medulla).

At each interface, the sound wave can be either **refracted** or **reflected**. **Refraction** happens when the sound wave is transmitted through the interface. Generally, the refracted angle is null. However, if multiple refractions happen, they can considerably damage the image.

The reflected wave is more interesting. There is **reflection** when the interface has a size equal to or bigger than the length of ultrasound waves used (the wave length is about 0.5 mm to 3.5 MHz and 0.2 mm to 7.5 MHz). When the interface size is smaller than the wavelength, it is called **scattering**. Indeed, when the wave bumps into a smooth and large surface, such as the gallbladder wall, the reflected angle is equal to the angle of incidence. On the contrary, if the surface is small (inferior to the wave length) and irregular, as in the hepatic parenchyma, the wave is divided into many smaller waves (scattered) and reflected in several directions. The reflected wave is essential to produce echographic images.

Indeed, the waves that are reflected toward the probe hit the piezoelectric crystal and the sound energy is converted into electrical energy, thanks to the crystal. Calculating the time used by the sound to go from the probe to the reflector and back, the echograph can know how far the reflector is. Likewise, the intensity of the reflected sound wave is used to calculate the reflecting power of the object. Every surrounding has a different spreading rate. The echograph calculator will use the average value of this rate (1540 m/s).

In order to avoid interferences between the emitted and reflected waves, ultrasounds are transmitted discontinuously (or in pulsed mode). The more the ultrasounds have to go far, the longer the time of emission and the lower the **pulse**

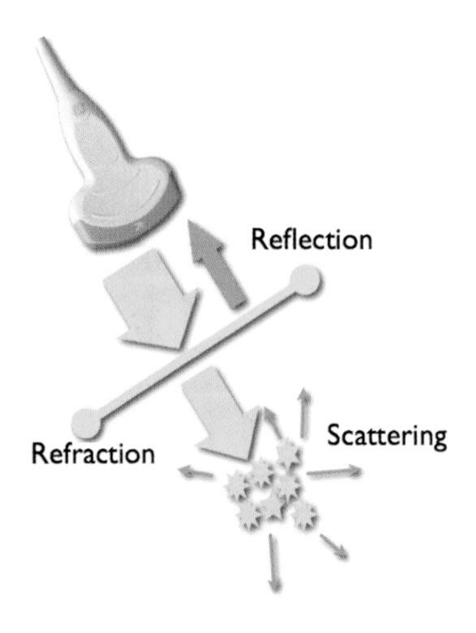

repetition frequency (PRF). Usually, the PRF is between 10 and 20 cycles per second (10–20 Hz). Each pulse produces a new image (frame), which is displayed on the screen as a real-time animated image.

The proportion of transmitted (refracted) or reflected sound while striking an interface depends on the difference in **acoustic impedance** between the tissues that constitute the interface. The acoustic impedance, measured in Rayl or Pascal second per meter is the product of the density of the tissue and the velocity with which it propagates sound. Most of tissues in the human body have quite similar impedance (see graph on page 14) and only a small proportion of sound is reflected. However, air and bones have very different values compared with other tissues. Therefore, when ultrasound collides with them, it is reflected. This implies that these interfaces appear with a greater intensity on the display screen and create a shadow behind them because the reflected sound can't reach deeper structures. The consequence is that ultrasound doesn't permit to see what is behind a bone or an air structure.

The use of gel prevents the creation of air pockets between the probe and the skin, which would provoke a total reflection of ultrasound.

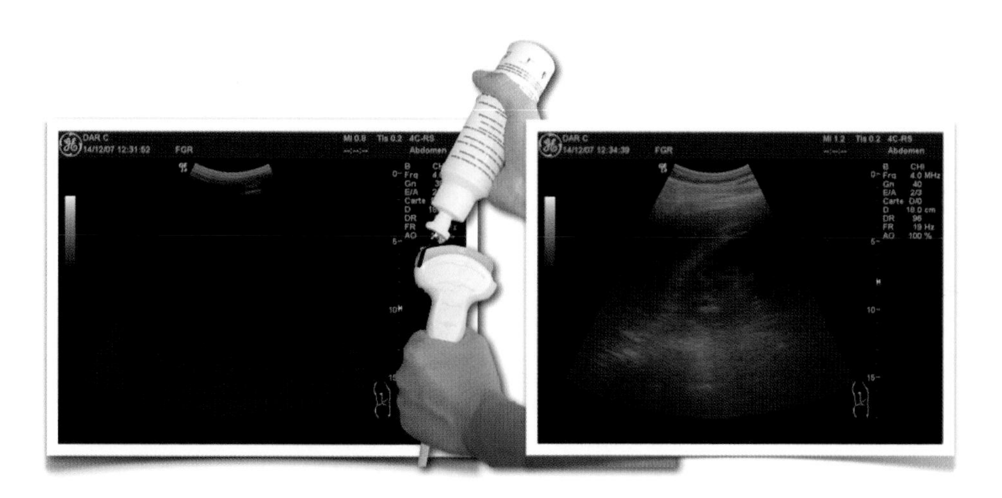

Image without gel

Image with gel

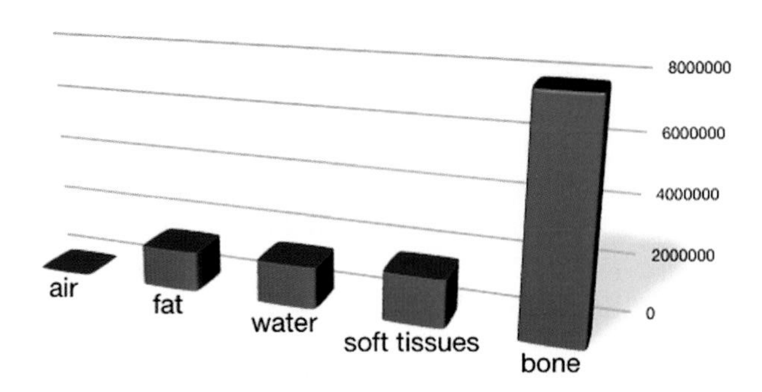

Resolution

Resolution is considered as the capacity to distinguish two different points. As far as echography machines are concerned, resolution can be measured on two bases: axial and lateral.

- **Axial resolution** is measured along the propagation axis of the sound wave. It is exactly proportional to the emission frequency of ultrasound.
- **Lateral resolution** is measured perpendicular to axial resolution. Lateral resolution depends on the probe design, especially on the number of piezoelectric crystals. It changes according to the width of the sector of image created and also depends on focusing. Axial resolution is always superior to lateral resolution.

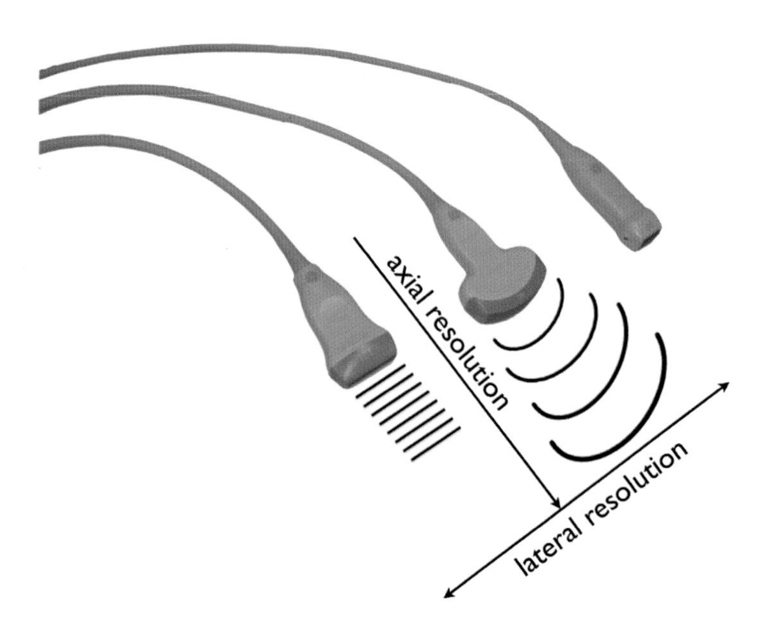

■ The probes

There are different sorts of echographic probes or transducers. Most of apparatuses have an abdominal curvilinear low-frequency transducer and a linear high-frequency transducer for vessels, nerves, and soft tissues. The former is wider and curved. The ultrasound beams are organized to create a "cone," the tip of which is the transducer. It permits to visualize wide parts of abdomen or pelvis. The usual frequency of this type of probe is between 2 and 5 MHz. The second probe, for soft parts, gives a rectangular image and its frequency is between 7.5 and 15 MHz depending on the models.

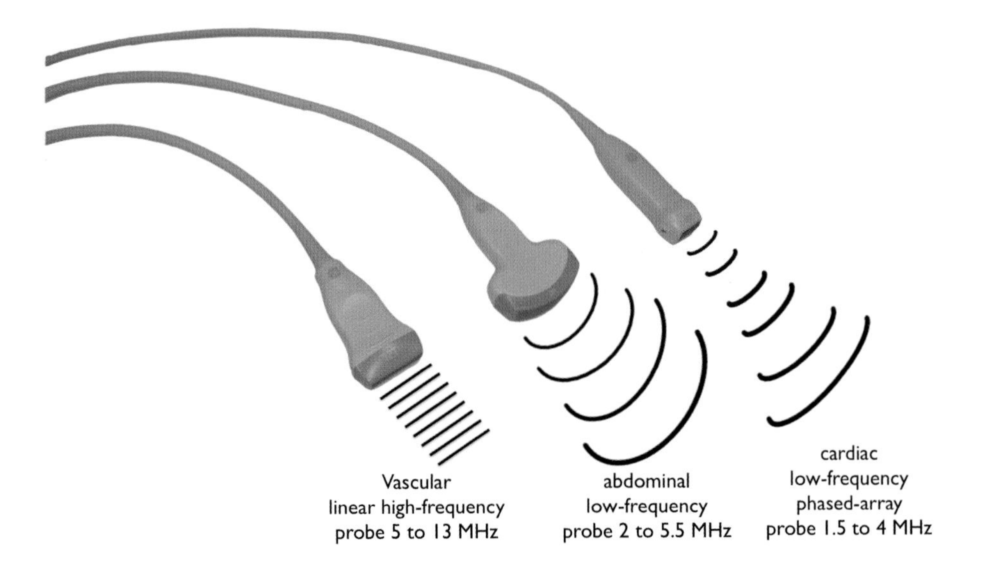

The frequency of emission of ultrasound is a compromise between resolution and penetration. We can obtain better-resolution images with high-frequency probes but the sound waves are absorbed more quickly when they go through tissues. A 10 MHz probe will not penetrate beyond 8 cm, while a 2 MHz will be able to penetrate 30 cm deep but with a reduced quality of resolution.

The technological evolution permitted to create multi-frequency probes that can produce, to a certain extent, different frequencies. For example, the low-frequency probes can use 2 to 5 MHz waves, and high-frequency probes can use 7.5 to 15 MHz waves. Thanks to this, we can adapt the probe settings according to the patient's morphology and the depth of the organ we examine.

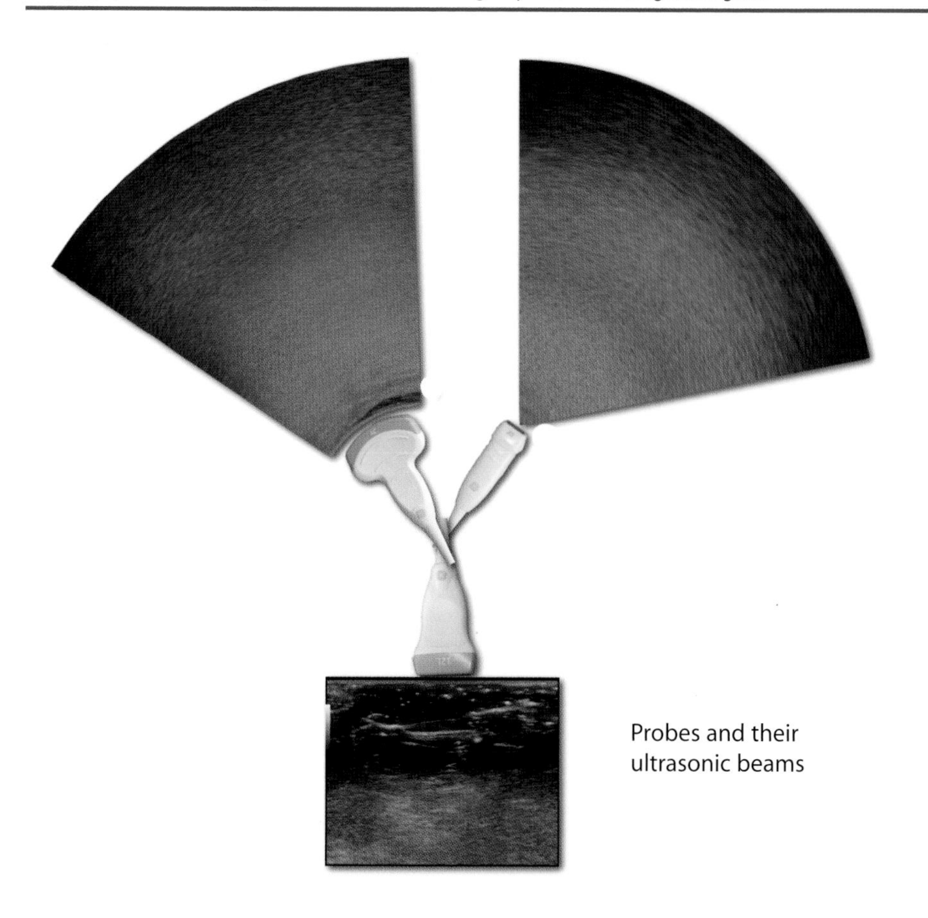

Probes and their ultrasonic beams

There are more specialized probes that answer to specific needs and permit to get closer to the organ you want to visualize (intracavity probe, transesophageal probe, endovascular probe).

■ The echogenicity of tissues

The interpretation of two-dimensional ultrasound images is based upon the observation of structures with a different echogenicity. **The echogenicity** of a tissue or interface is its capacity to generate an echo.

We can distinguish three types of basic echoes (from black to white):

- The **anechogenic** structures (black) don't produce echoes and correspond to liquids (urine, bile, blood, effusions). They appear black on the display screen.
- The **structure echoes** (all gray variations) are composed of low amplitude that corresponds to a diffuse reflection and an ultrasound scattering in relatively homogeneous surroundings. These structure echoes represent the essential part of the echographic image and permit to image the parenchymatous organs on a "tissue scale." We distinguish **hypoechogenic** structures, which appear rather dark (dark

gray), and **hyperechogenic** structures, which are the origin of numerous reflections of ultrasound and make a clear image on the screen. The notion of hypo- or hyper-echogenic is relative according to surrounding structures. The hepatic parenchyma is generally darker because it is hypoechogenic, compared to the spleen parenchyma, which is hyperechogenic. When two structures have the same echogenicity, we call them isoechogenic.
- The **interface echoes** (white) show the juxtaposition of soft tissues and air or of soft tissues and a hard, mineralized, or metallic structure. In the body, the diaphragm, the bones, the digestive air, and pulmonary air make very marked interface echoes.

The echogenicity of a tissue depends mainly on its homogeneity, vascularization, fat content and fibrous tissue content.

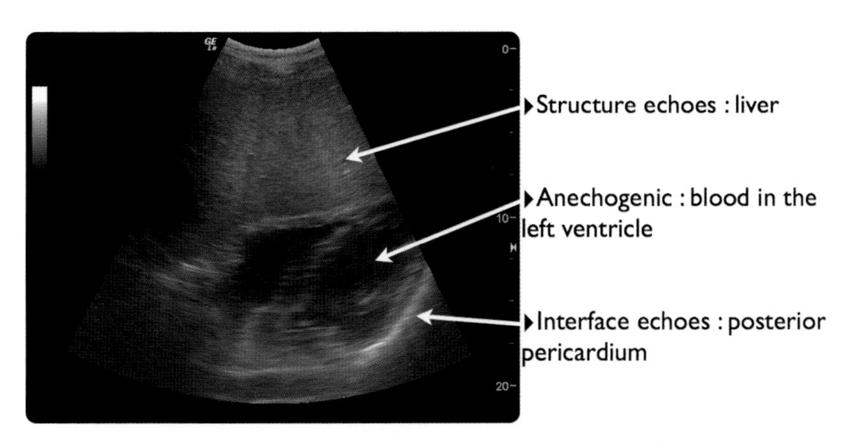

Subcostal view of the heart

Artifacts

(Novices can skip this part and come back to it later. They will not hesitate to complete their knowledge, thanks to specialized books.)

Echography image artifacts are echoes that don't correspond to an anatomic structure. Artifacts are the unavoidable consequence of interaction between the ultrasonic beam, the tissues and the computing material of the echograph. Thus, it is important to know them in order to identify them and make arrangements if possible.

Noise

It is constituted by granular echoes, particularly in cystic areas. It is caused by an excessive gain in the near field. We can reduce it by diminishing the gain setting.

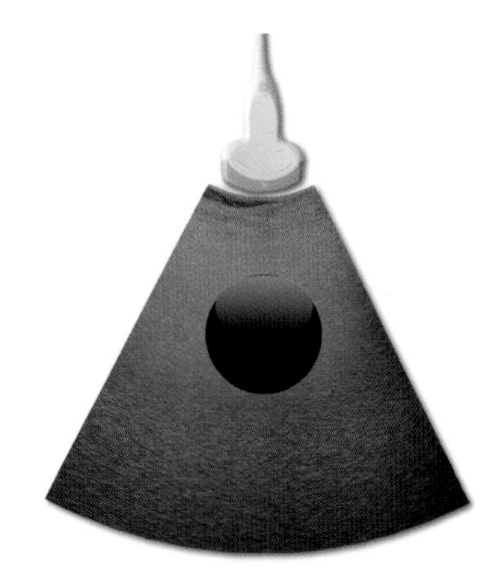

Posterior reinforcement and acoustic shadowing

When ultrasound goes through a not much reflecting area, the deeper structures are hit by ultrasonic waves that produce a higher reflection. This phenomenon is known as posterior reinforcement. It is usually found with liquid structures such as cysts and can be useful in differential diagnoses with solid structures.

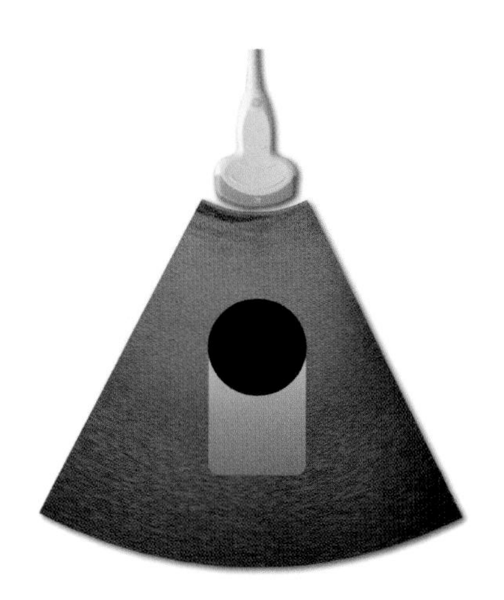

On the contrary, when the ultrasound beam collides with a strongly reflective interface, for example a gallstone, most of it is reflected. Thus, the object creates a shadow with a black line behind itself; this is called acoustic shadowing, which can be particularly useful to detect smaller stones because the shadow cone can often be better observed than the object that creates it.

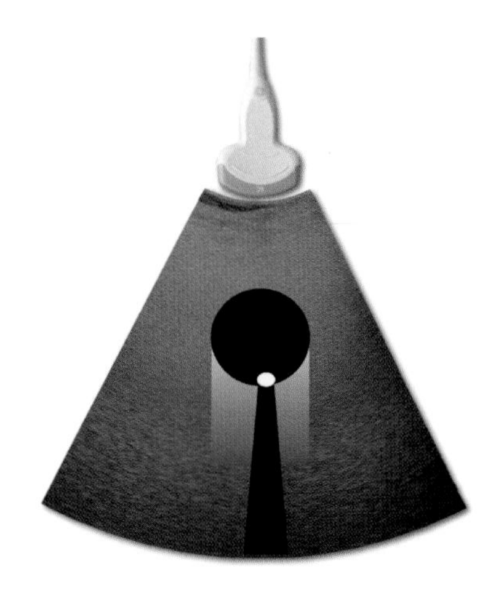

Reverberation
Parallel echo bands are separated by regular intervals. The reverberations occur on interfaces between adjacent surroundings that have very different acoustic impedances. The ultrasound waves are partially reflected by the second interface and some of these echoes are again reflected by the posterior part of the first interface. This is how a repetitive back-and-forth movement of reflections occurs, and they appear as distinct parallel bands or very intense reflectors with a very narrow trail like a comet tail.

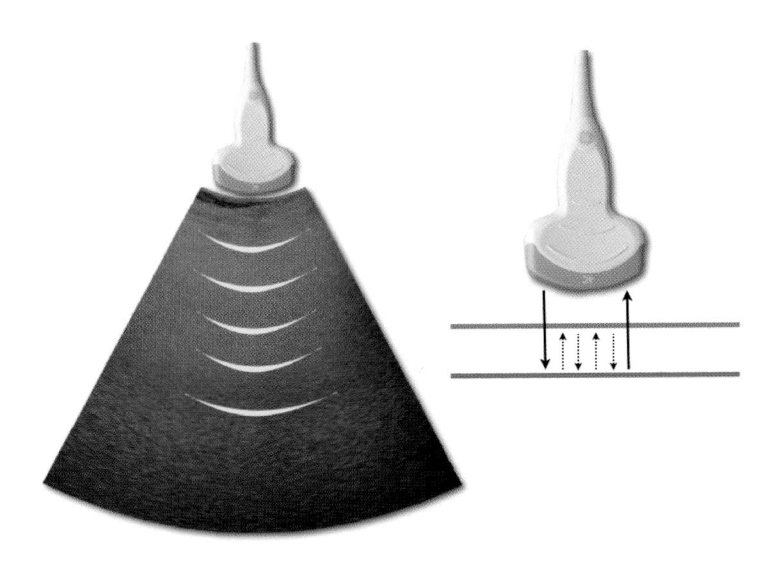

Artifact due to the beam width
It appears as a group of thin granular echoes dispersed along the inner part of cystic structures when their wall is struck diagonally by the ultrasound beam. The main beam emitted by the transducer has a defined width and, when it strikes a sidelong interface, it goes at the same time through the echo-free inner part of the cyst and through its very reflective wall. The echogenicity of these different structures is averaged in order to provide an image, and this gives the impression that blurred echoes cover the cyst wall.

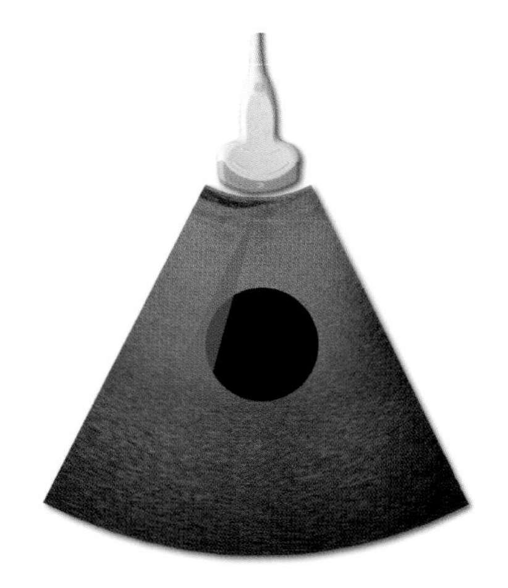

Mirror image

A mirror image artifact is the virtual image of a real object that is formed behind a very reflective interface. It is caused by the reflection of the beam at the level of the "supposed" reflector. The virtual image appears behind the interface on the way of the main beam. The diaphragm is an excellent reflector of hepatic structures.

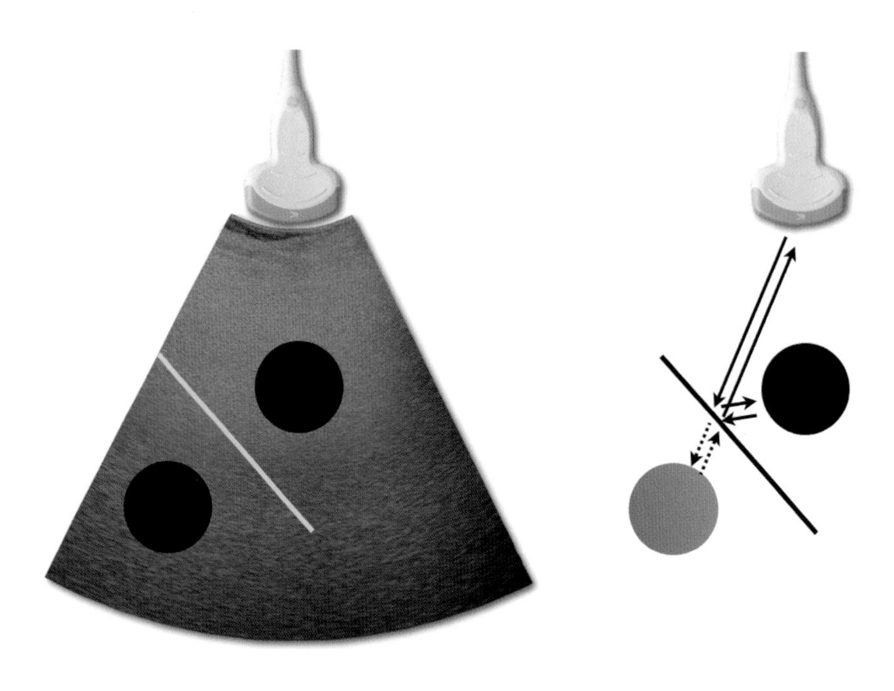

Edge shadow

An edge shadow is a thin acoustic shadow that appears just behind the lateral edges of a cystic structure. It is caused by refraction and the propagation of sound that reaches the cystic wall with a tangential angle. Since its energy vanishes, the sound doesn't spread in deeper levels and an acoustic shadow appears.

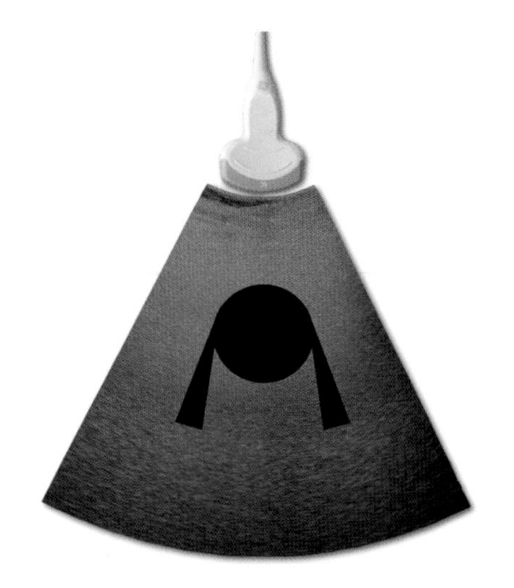

Anisotropy

The echogenicity of certain structures, known as anisotropic, depends on the direction of the ultrasound beam. We notice a variation of the echogenicity according to the direction of ultrasound. The echogenicity is at its maximum when the ultrasound is directed perpendicular to the reflective surface and diminishes when the reflection is sidelong. The bigger the obliqueness angle, the less echogenic seems the structure. The best example is a tendinous echography for which echogenicity strongly depends on the position of the probe. **The echogenicity is at its maximum when the tendon is perpendicular to the probe.** This artifact sets the use of linear probes for the examination of tendons. The nerves, less sensitive to this phenomenon, seem to light up when the tendons and muscles disappear, that is to say when the ultrasound beam is leaned.

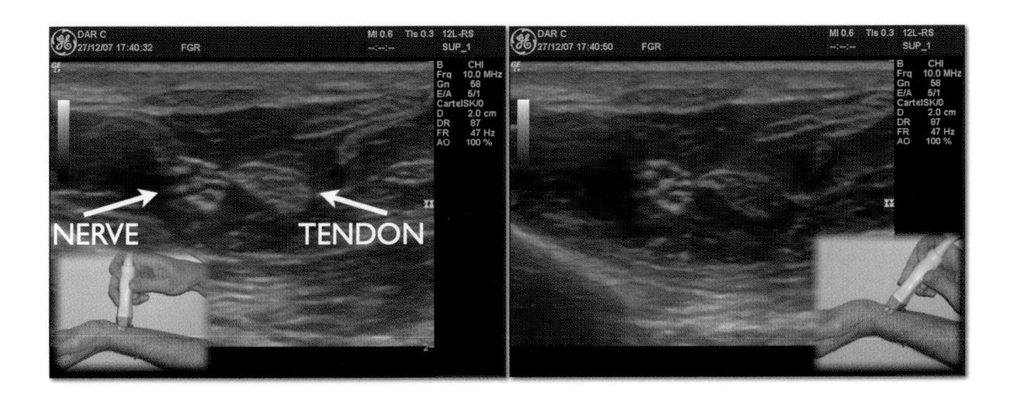

■ The echograph users' manual *(Machine settings)*

The most difficult part, when we are in front of the machine, is to plug the socket in and find the on/off switch. The rest, as you will see later, is logical.

The echographs, as real computers, are sensitive to untimely unplugging, which cause the destruction of the hard drive. To avoid this, the on/off switch was often set in an inaccessible place. Now it gradually changes with the arrival of laptops, which have a battery that prevents any sudden stop of power supply.

The echographs that we call "button box" are provided along with a considerable number of options so that the user can modify at will the echographic image obtained. Let's see how switches permit to do the essential settings for a first use.

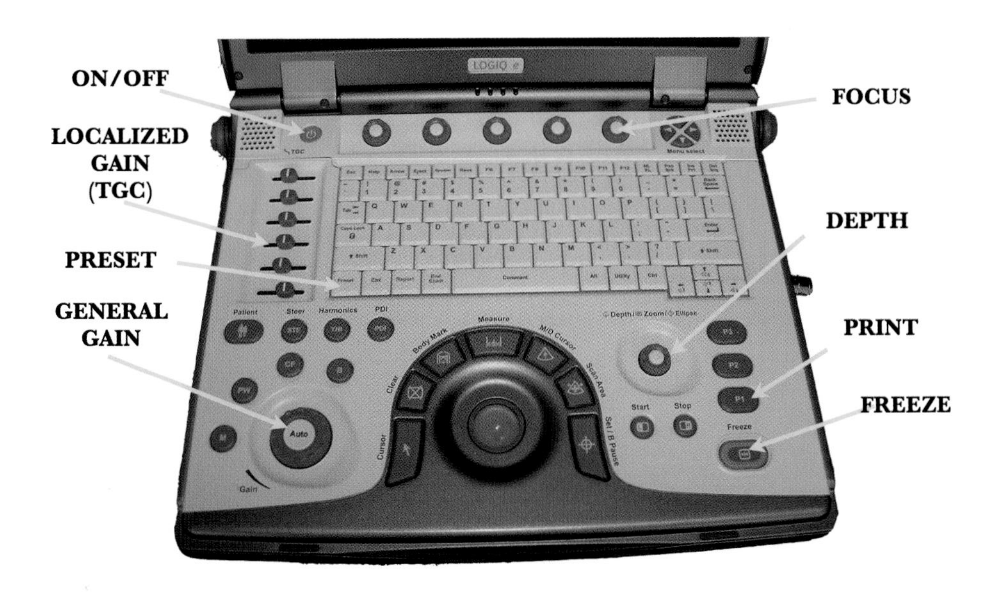

Choosing the probe

Choosing the probe will depend on the organ to be examined. A superficial echography will need a high-frequency probe, while the echography of a deep organ will need a low-frequency probe. In the case of a multi-frequency probe, the frequency will be set the best way according to the patient's morphology as well as the depth of the organ examined in order to obtain the best possible quality of image.

It is generally possible to choose these settings, thanks to the "PROBE" switch. The apparatus displays the available probes, and you have to choose one. On mobile machines, once the probe is connected to the computer, everything is automatically configured. It is also possible, thanks to the 'PRESET' menu, to choose the probe with a special presetting for the organ you want to visualize.

Depth

The operator can choose the depth of ultrasound exploration, thus changing the tissues displayed on the screen. This is important to optimize the image. Because of the time necessary for ultrasounds to cover in both directions the distance between the probe and the object to be visualized, the deeper the exploration, the lower the image display frequency (frame). Moreover, the structures that are explored will be displayed in a smaller size on the screen. On the contrary, if the exploration depth is too low, parts of the structure to be visualized will not appear within the frame. In practice, from the initial setting, we can change the depth in order to obtain, if possible, the most entire display of the explored organ.

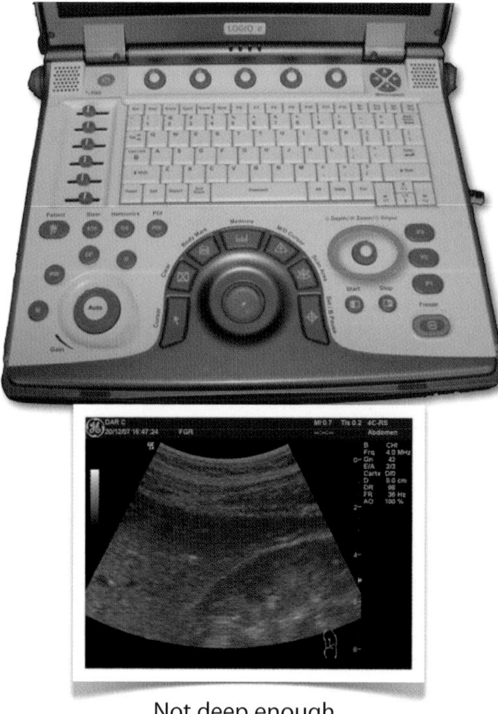

Not deep enough

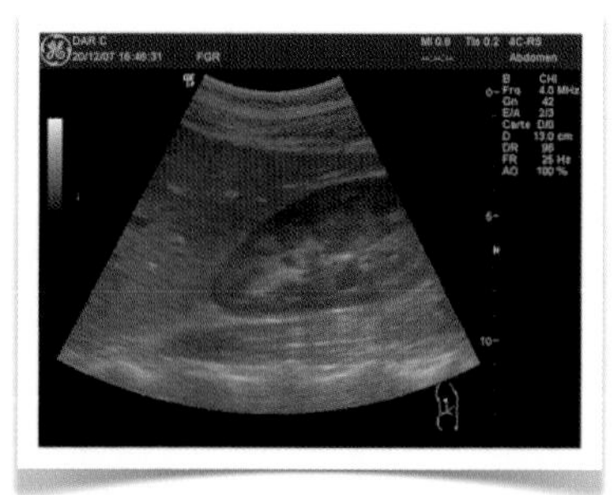

Good setting

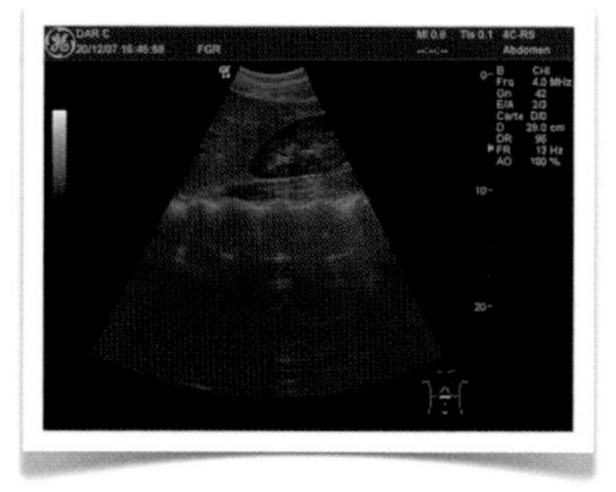

Too deep

Focus

As the edges of the ultrasound beam are not parallel, the beam converges to a focusing area. Beyond this area, the beam diverges. The depth and the size of the focusing area can be changed and are displayed, thanks to marks on the right side of the image on the screen. For an optimal image, the focusing area must be set so that it includes the whole anatomic part you want to explore.

Gain

The gain, or signal amplification, can be set in two different ways.

1. The general gain produces an amplification of signal that comes back to the probe, whatever its origin. Thus, the enhancement of general gain increases the amplitude of signals coming from distant structures as well as from structures near the probe. Usually the general gain is controlled with a knob.

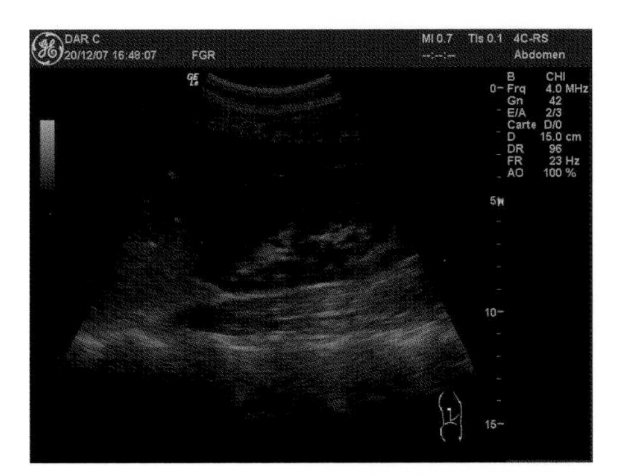

Not enough gain

Too much gain

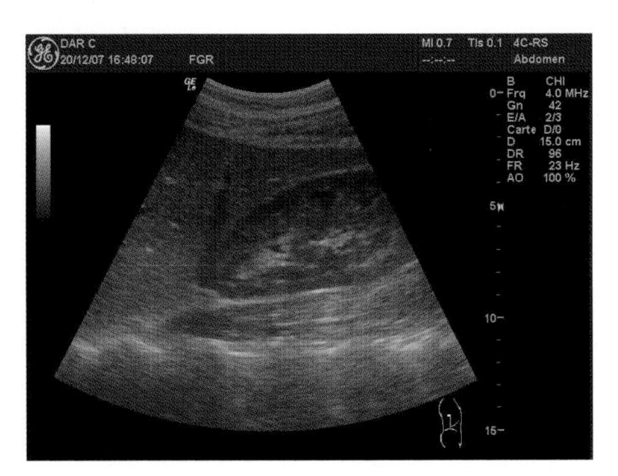

Good setting

2. The localized gain, thanks to time gain compensation (TGC), permits the operator to amplify the signals coming from different depths. Thus, we can obtain a more homogeneous image, thanks to the amplification of distant structures for which attenuation is more important due to the distance to cover.

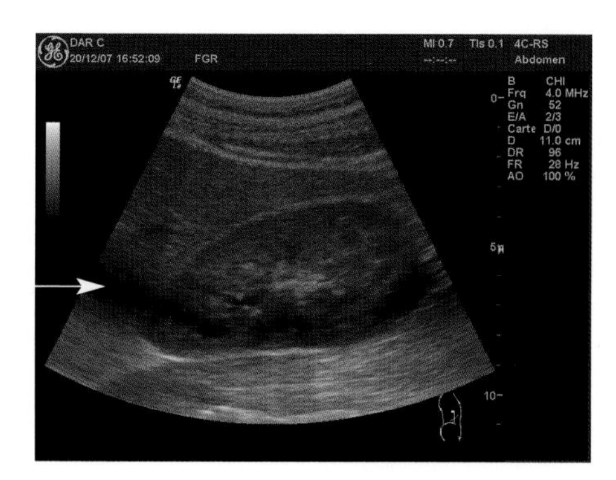

Not enough gain

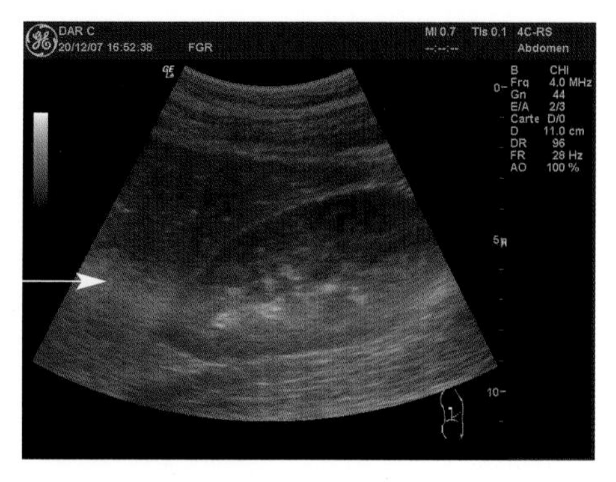

Too much gain

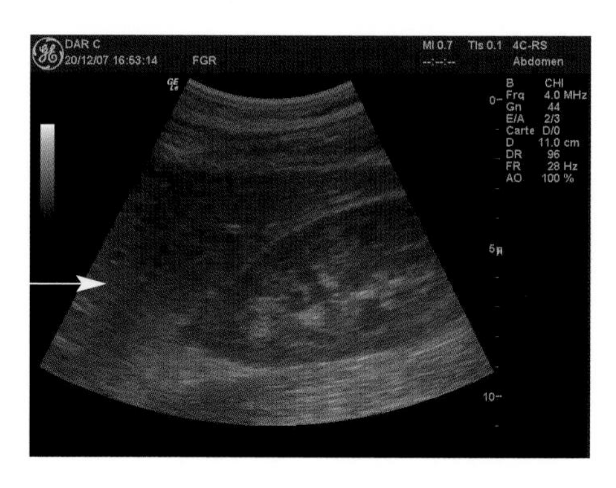

Good setting

Freeze

It permits to freeze the image in order to put a comment, to measure something, and then to store or print it, or to quietly watch it on the screen, all this releasing the probe.

Print

This switch permits to print the image if a printer is connected to the echograph.

Here is, briefly, what is essential to know to be able to use an echograph in anesthesiology and to obtain images according to the organs wanted.

■ Application

Thinking of all these gray shades and not seeing the point of this machine, I tidied it in a corner, put a dust cover on it, and promised myself they wouldn't catch me again on that.

This way, please!

"I want my local, I want my local." The sentence was so repeated that I thought I was hearing the latest fashionable hit when I entered into the preanesthesia room. Seeing the nurse's face, I quickly understood that the nice lady, wearing a bouffant cap that hid her superb hairstyle, had not been premedicated enough. I pretended to be an outsider in the operating room, but I was quickly spotted and forced to participate in the turmoil. As she had to undergo the replacement of her left knee, she claimed for the block of the femoral nerve that my predecessor had promised her as a post-operatory analgesia, not to forget the tubing coming along with it. With zeal, I assured her that we would do it immediately. But once on the premises, it became really tricky because of the woman's plumpness, and I had difficulty to locate the target area. My fingers were deaf and blind. All self-confident, with a complacent smile, the nurse moved the echographic machine toward me.

As I had to look for the femoral nerve just beside the vessels, at a depth of less than 7 centimeters (at least I hoped so), I put the high-frequency linear probe into place, transversally on the groin so that the ultrasound beam went through the artery and the femoral vein, and made me notice two anechogenic areas (in black). Mobilizing the probe, along the limb root, I found the femoral vessels, circular, black, beating areas. I adjusted the depth, gain, and focus instinctively in order to have the best image of the area.

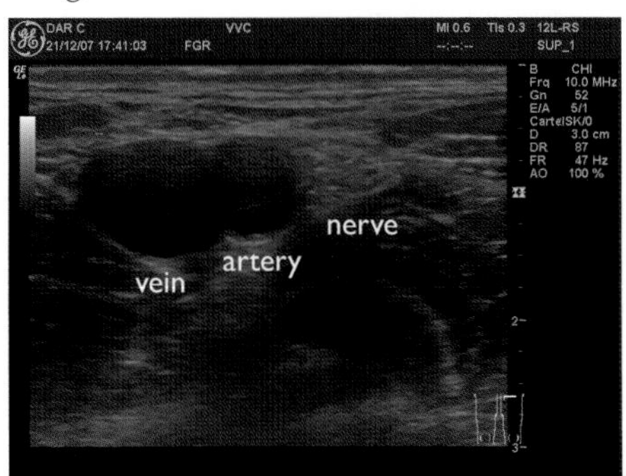

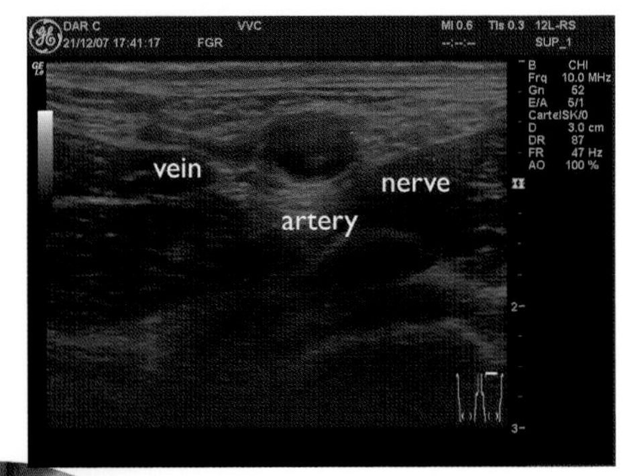

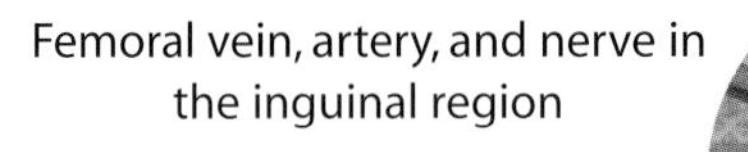
Femoral vein, artery, and nerve in the inguinal region

Disappearance of femoral vein when pushing

When I pushed softly the probe on the skin, I noticed that the vein was flattened and the artery remained clearly visible. With the artery located, I leaned the transducer, looked 1 centimeter further, and observed the appearance of a more brilliant structure: the crural nerve. I made the probe slide and carefully put the nerve in the middle of the screen. I marked the skin where the middle of the transducer was and located the depth of the nerve on the side of the screen. Then, I put down the probe. After having meticulously disinfected the skin, I took the needle with the neurostimulator and stung on the mark, gently pushing the needle in. When I reached the indicated depth, the patient's kneecap began to convulse at the rhythm of electricity. Pleased with myself, I finished the procedure under the approving eye of my patient, who at last had her tubing!

I had just found a purpose for the technological jumble.

In echography, the peripheral nerve is a fibrillar structure, striped in the longitudinal section and oval-shaped in the transverse section. It is made of hypoechogenic fascicles (black) in hyperechogenic surroundings (white). The nerve is not very prone to anisotropy and is very flexible when the transducer pushes on it. It progresses between the muscle compartments, often with the vessels, or within ducts. The proximity of vessels is very helpful because they are easy to find in B-mode (the basic mode), especially thanks to color Doppler.

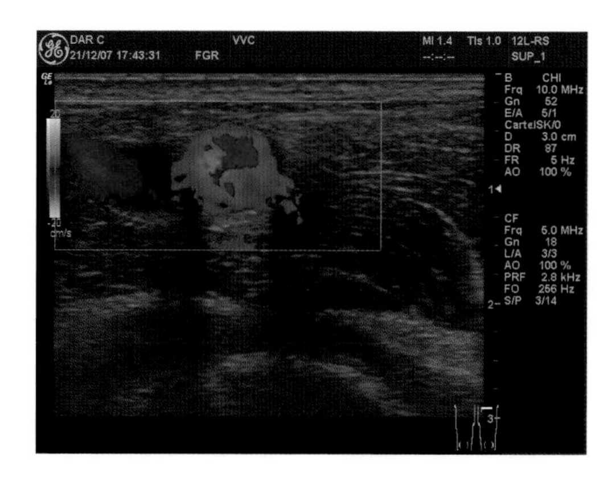

Femoral vein and artery in color Doppler

The nerve can be visualized in its short axis (transverse view) or its long axis (longitudinal view).

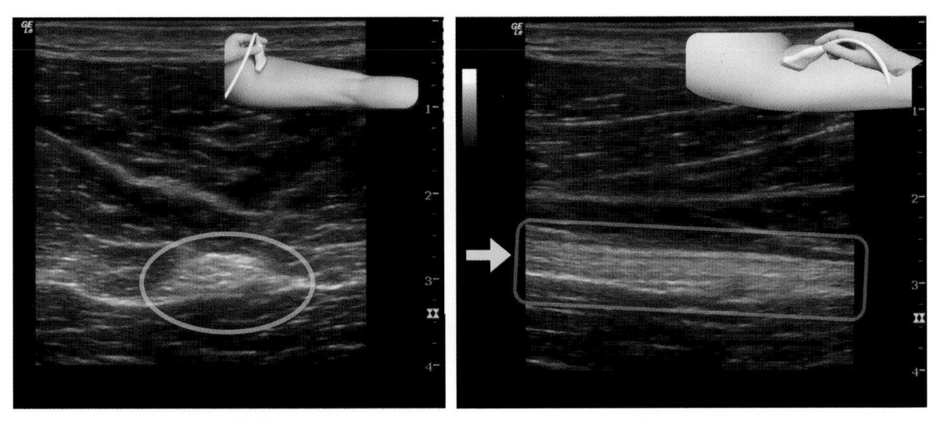

Transverse view
of the sciatic nerve

Longitudinal view
of the sciatic nerve

There are two common needle insertion approaches:

In-plane needle approach:

The needle is placed in line with and parallel to the transducer. Both the needle shaft and tip are visualized. In theory, needle-to-nerve contact can be followed in real time.

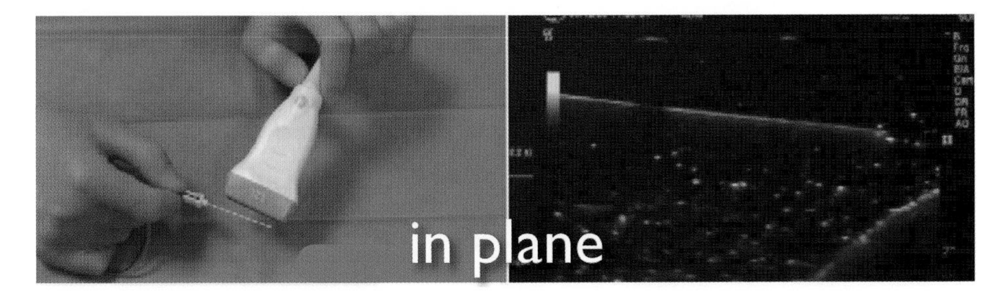

Out-of-plane needle approach:

The needle is placed perpendicular to the transducer. The needle shaft and tip are visualized as a hyperechoic dot on ultrasound. In this case, needle, nerve, and tissue movements are observed. The needle tip may be difficult to locate accurately. Actual needle-to-nerve contact can be confirmed by nerve stimulation and local anesthetic spread pattern (hydro-location).

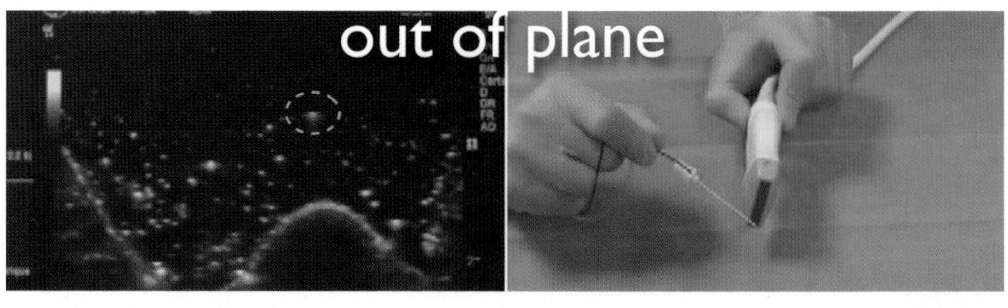

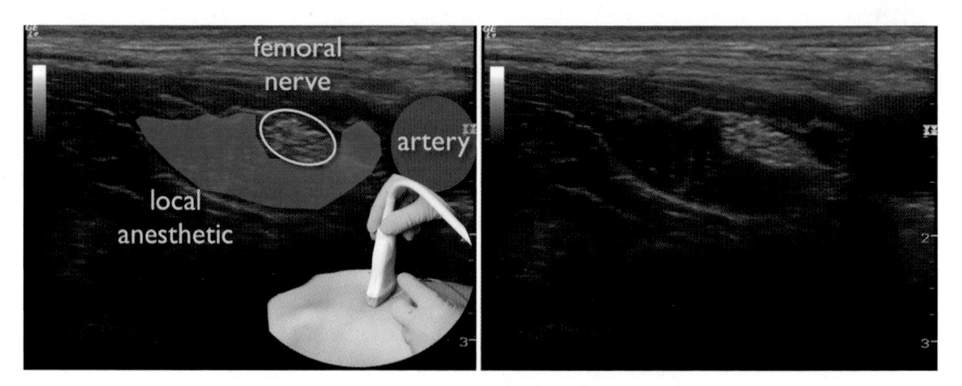

Femoral nerve blockade (out of plane)

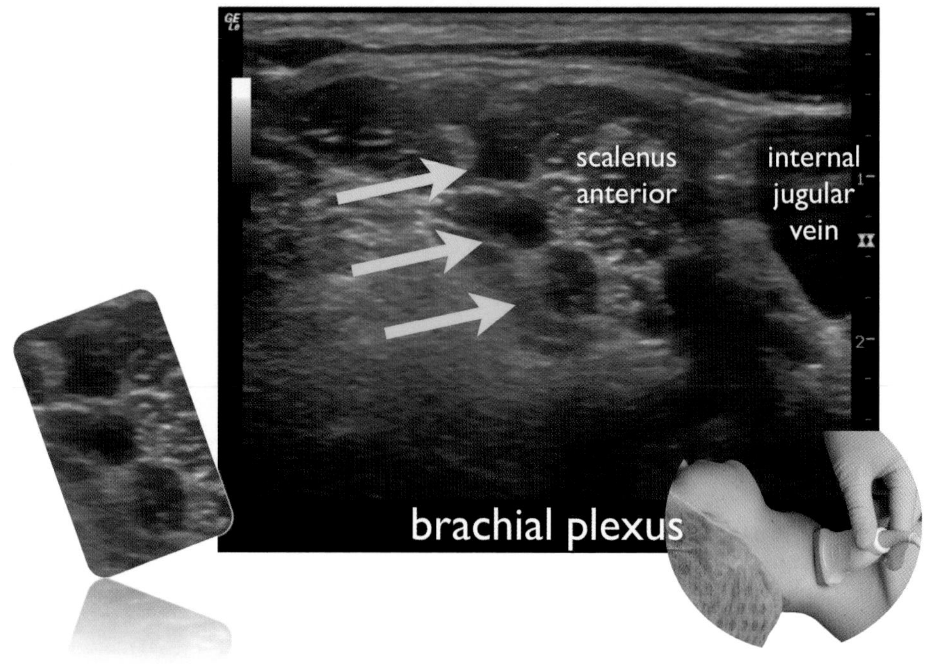

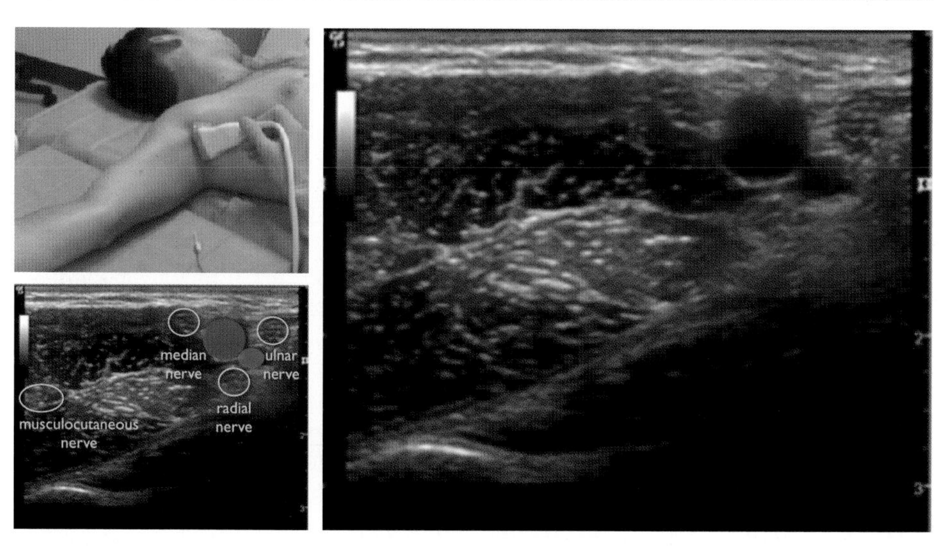

Sono anatomy of the braxial plexus

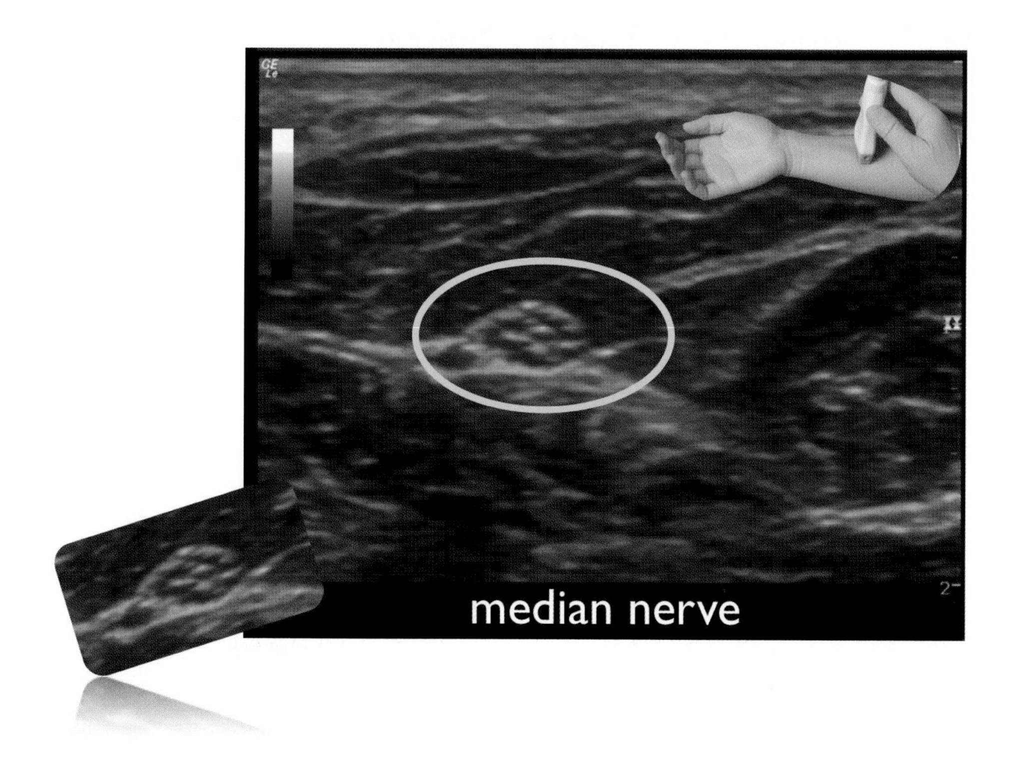

Details of industry

The nice salesman, filled with remorse as he had abandoned me, kindly sent me the following details about B-mode and color mode.

B-mode

In B-mode, the most common, each echo is represented by a light point (brightness) along the base line (ultrasonic beam). As a result, a line of more or less bright points appears. When we do the scanning of the ultrasonic beam, we obtain a two-dimensional (2D) image. Generally, the scanning is electronic. It can also be mechanical according to the type of probe.

The brightness range is divided into several gray levels (256 levels in average). This way we obtain an echographic image that will represent a section of the body where the most brilliant points in the image correspond to the most ultrasound reflecting structures, that is the most echogenic structures.

As for the echographic representation of a vessel in B-mode, the bloodstream will be seen as a black area surrounded by white lines in a longitudinal section and white circles in a transverse section.

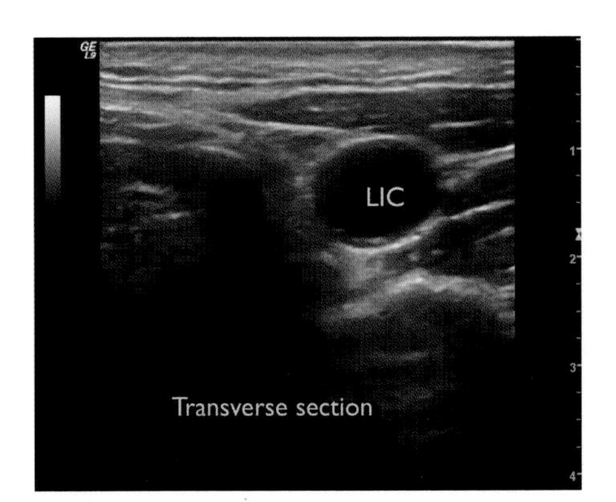

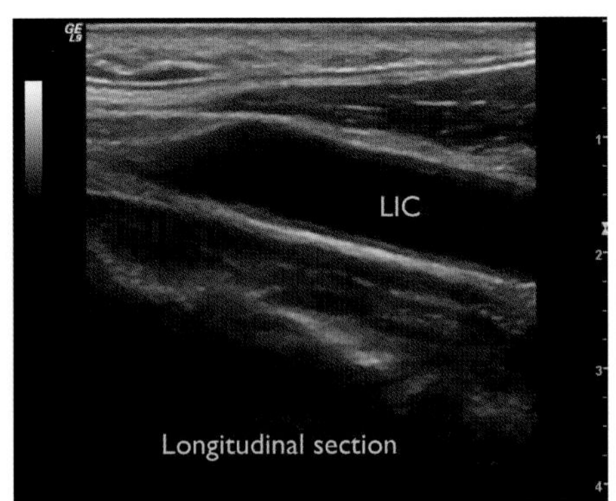

Images of the left internal carotid

The main parameters of B-mode settings are as follows:

- The depth of the exploration field according to the position of the organ you must see (superficial or deep).
- The gain, in order to adapt the image to the visualization and thus have a good uniformity from surface to depth. Generally speaking, there are two gains: the total gain, which acts upon the whole image, and the TGC gain, made of several linear potentiometers, each of them related to an area of the image.
- Focusing consists in displaying on the screen the area that we most want to observe, with the best definition. Usually, it is an index (a little triangle, for example) on the right or the left of the image that we can move from the surface to the depth of the image and inversely. For special studies, it is possible to increase the number of indexes and thus to widen the maximal definition area.

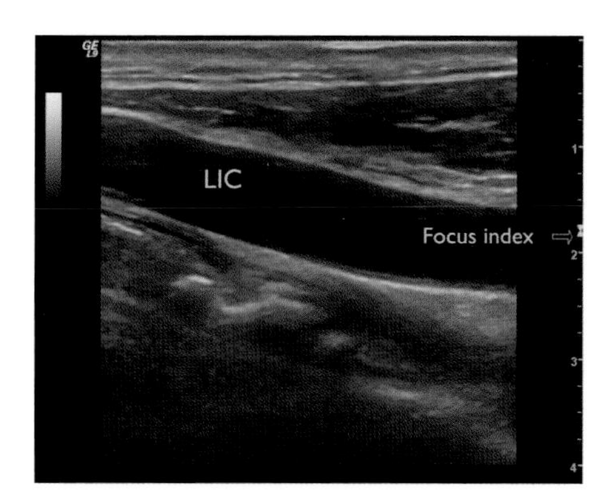

- In an echograph, other settings are possible within the B-mode. They will be used during the installation with the application engineer, in order to help you to obtain the image you want, and to save them so that you can automatically enjoy the settings each time you use the echograph.
- Some of the latest-generation echographs have one only button that automatically optimizes the image, thanks to a pulse.

The color Doppler mode

In the eighties, with a view to improve the display of an echographic image, the color Doppler mode was introduced. The process consists in coloring the inner parts of a vessel.

Two colors were chosen: red and blue, in order to see the direction of circulation in the vessel. This is how a color scale was created: dark colors for slow velocities and light colors for high velocities.

The transition from red to blue occurs in a black area that represents a nonexistent velocity. Moreover, in order to display the turbulences, some colored curves can even have a green shade. Several types of color scales are available on echographs.

An agreement was reached: any bloodstream that moves toward the transducer will be in red. Any bloodstream that moves away rom the transducer will be in blue.

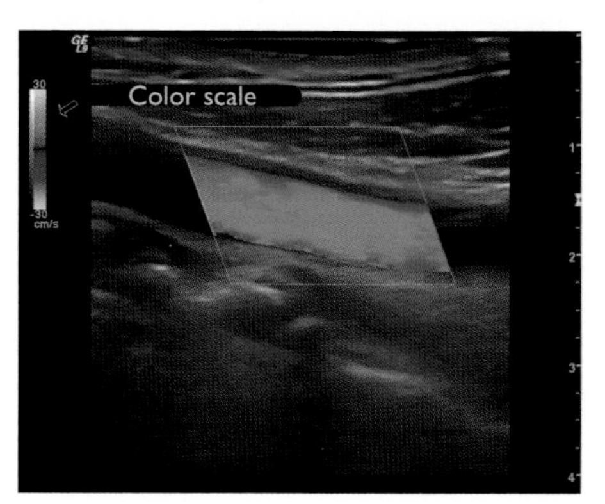

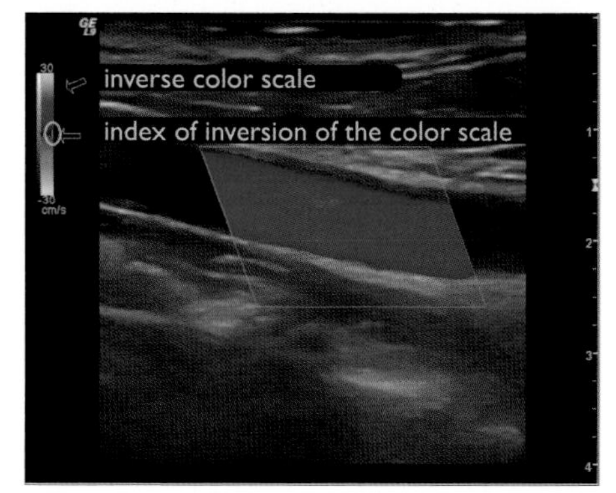

Nevertheless, we have to take much care about the interpretation of the bloodstream direction on an image. Indeed, all the latest-generation echographs have an inversion button. As a consequence, we must always take into account the color scale displayed on the screen. The color that is higher on the color scale will always correspond to the circulation toward the transducer.

As color Doppler mode is always used after a first visualization in B-mode, we will consider that the image is already well set up. To activate the color Doppler mode, you have to find the COLOR FLOW (CF) button and push it. Here are the main setting parameters in color Doppler mode:

Pulse Repetition Frequency (PRF) setting is very important. Indeed, it is necessary to fit the velocity of detection of the echograph to the velocity of circulation of the vessel you want to observe. If the detection velocity is inferior to the real red cell circulation velocity in the vessel, too many colors are displayed on the screen, with successive and untimely changes from red to blue and vice versa. We call this phenomenon "aliasing" or frequential ambiguity: "the machine doesn't know anymore what it is analyzing."

Otherwise, if the detection velocity is superior to the real velocity, it is difficult, not to say impossible, to fill the vessel.

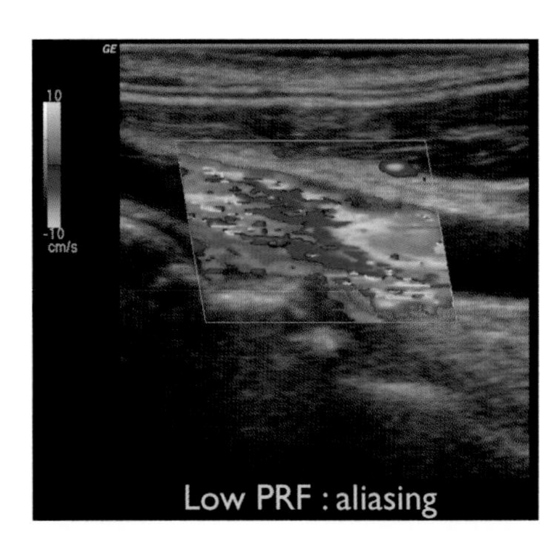

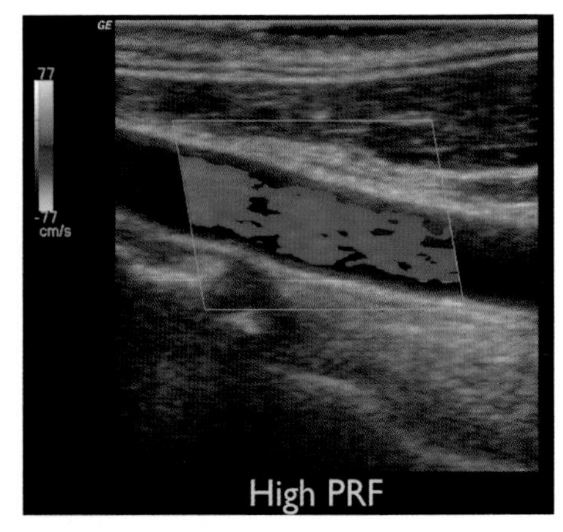

The gain setting is very important because it is the setting that will permit a good color filling of the vessel. Indeed, if the gain of the color is too high, the color bleeds outside the vessel walls; we talk about blooming. On the contrary, if the color gain is too low, only the center part of the vessel will be colored. A good image will display a color that perfectly follows the vessel walls.

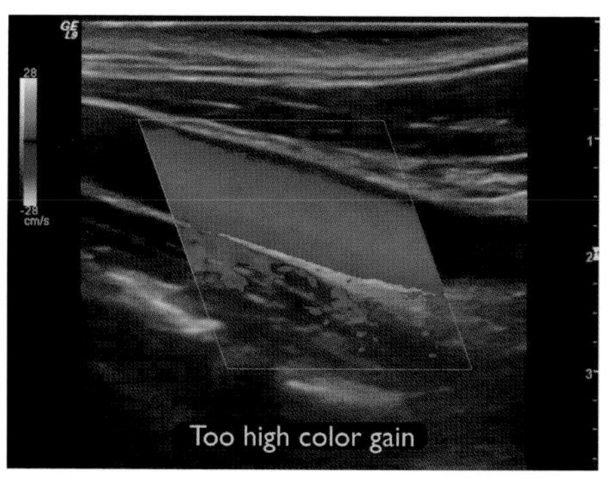

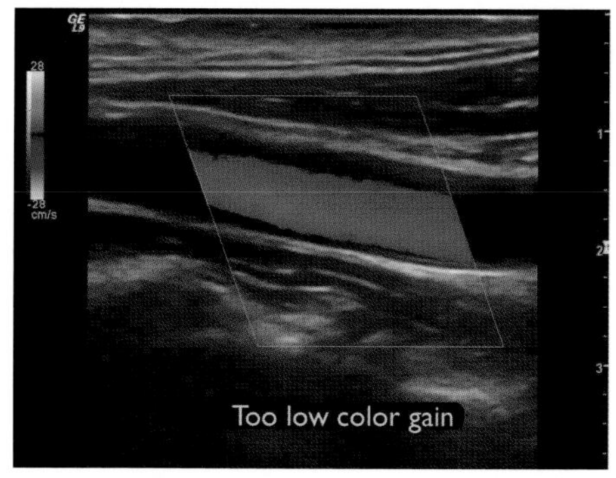

The size of the color box can be set up in order to visualize as well as possible the interesting area. Generally speaking, we can set it up in height and width. It's only in this area that any bloodstream will be represented in color.

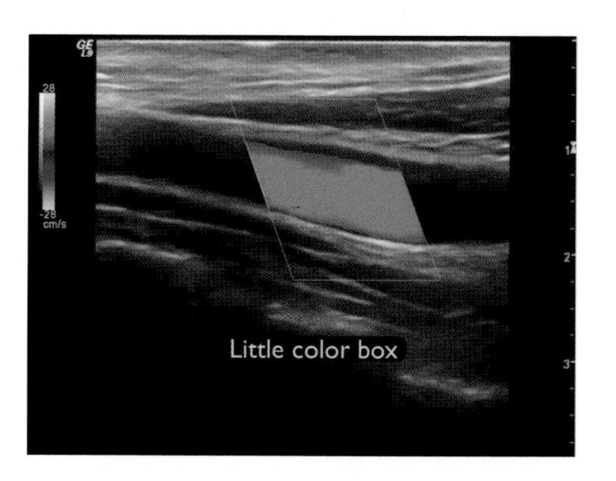

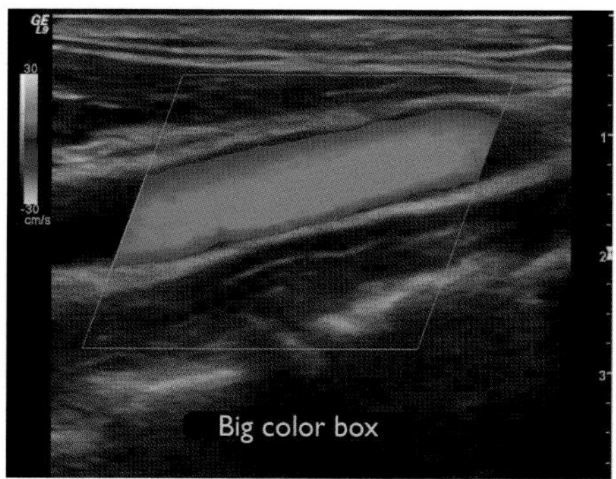

Inclination of the color box with the linear probes: in Doppler mode, the quality of image depends on the cosine a, where a is the angle between the axis of the probe and the axis of the cut vessel. If the vessel axis is parallel to the probe surface, the ultrasound beam is perpendicular to the vessel ($\alpha = 90°$, $\cos \alpha = 0$). As a consequence, there is no Doppler effect and the vessel will not be colored. In order to make up for this fact, we can lean the Doppler axis to the right or to the left. This creates an angle between the vessel axis and the probe surface, and thus allows the color filling of the examined vessel.

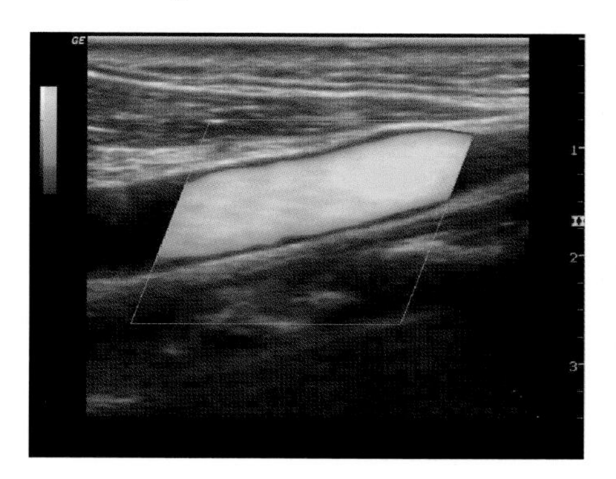

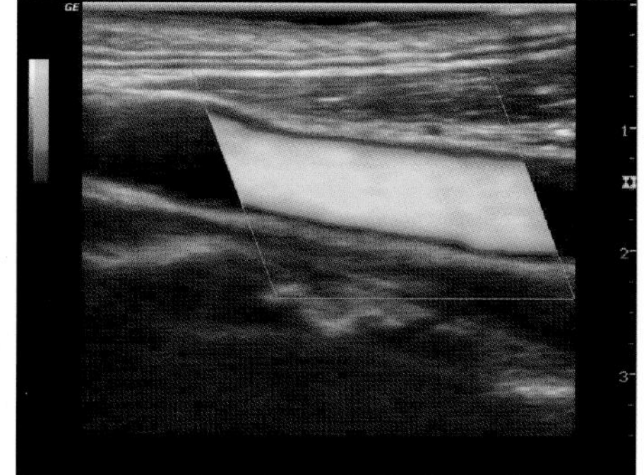

As for the B-mode, we can also set up other parameters in Doppler mode. They will be used during the installation with the application engineer, in order to help you to obtain the image you want, and then to save them.

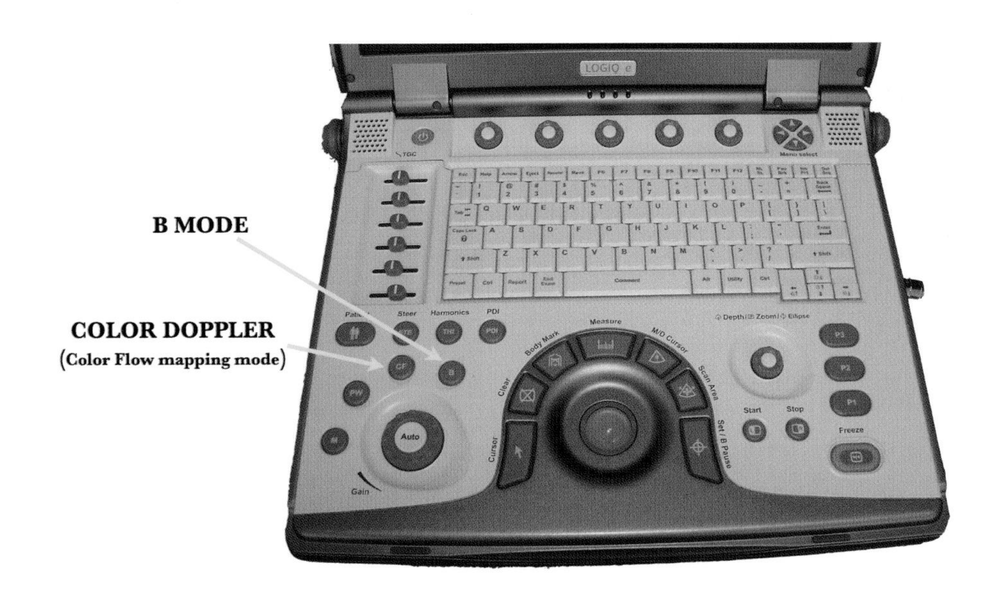

The doctor and the machine in front of the patient

■ Users' manual of the probe

Follow the **GPS** (the General Placed on the Side of the probe):

Encouraged by this first use, I promised myself to go into detail and no longer think of this technological jumble as a collection of lifeless parts but rather as an occasional help to complete my capacity to think, thanks to a complementary intern vision. (Oh, it even makes us philosophers!) In spite of these good intentions, I realized I was lost in space, and had difficulty to get my bearings on the screen.

Top and bottom

I easily understood that the top of the screen represents the beginning of the ultrasonic beam and the bottom of the screen represents the end of the ultrasonographic exploration, which depends on the ultrasound frequency and the depth setting you have chosen. The depth is displayed as a scale on the right side of the screen. As a rule between us, we'll define the sides of the screen according to the side of the operator face to the screen: the right hand of the operator touches the right side of the screen, and the left hand touches the left side.

Thus, the top of the screen represents the skin of the patient and the bottom the depth.

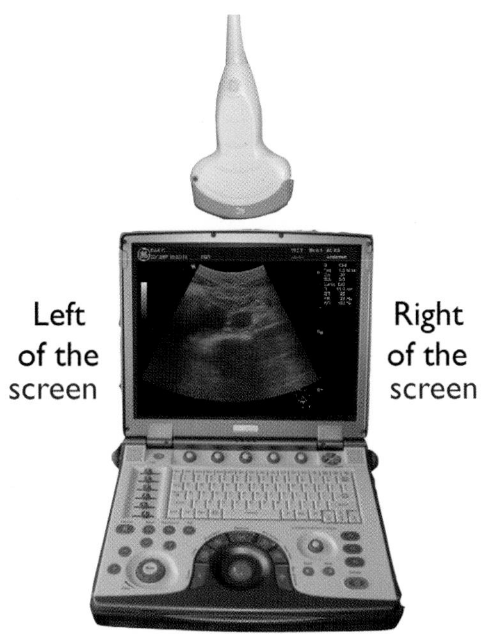

Right and left

And now, what are the right and left of the screen? Actually, the general decides! On one side of every transducer, there is a luminous mark, a notch, or a little raised pattern that corresponds to a logo placed on the top of the screen, on a specific side. For our machine, it is GE for GENERAL EL... (no advertising); for HP the pattern is HP; for others like SonoSite, it's a white point. To get one's bearings, we have to find the mark on the probe, and the logo on the screen, because both represent the same side of the ultrasonic beam.

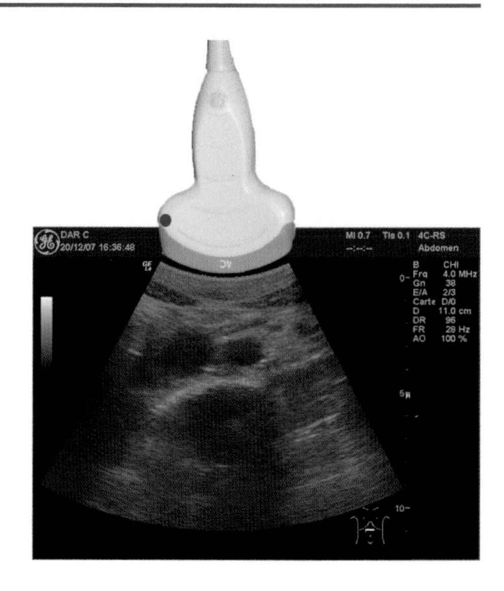

The sections

For us beginners, in order to progress in echography, there are two types of sections from which we can create all the intermediaries manipulating the probe. They are the transverse section and the longitudinal section. The transverse section goes from right to left and thus separates the head from feet, while the longitudinal section goes from head to feet separating the right and left sides. In both cases, the probe is held perpendicular to the skin.

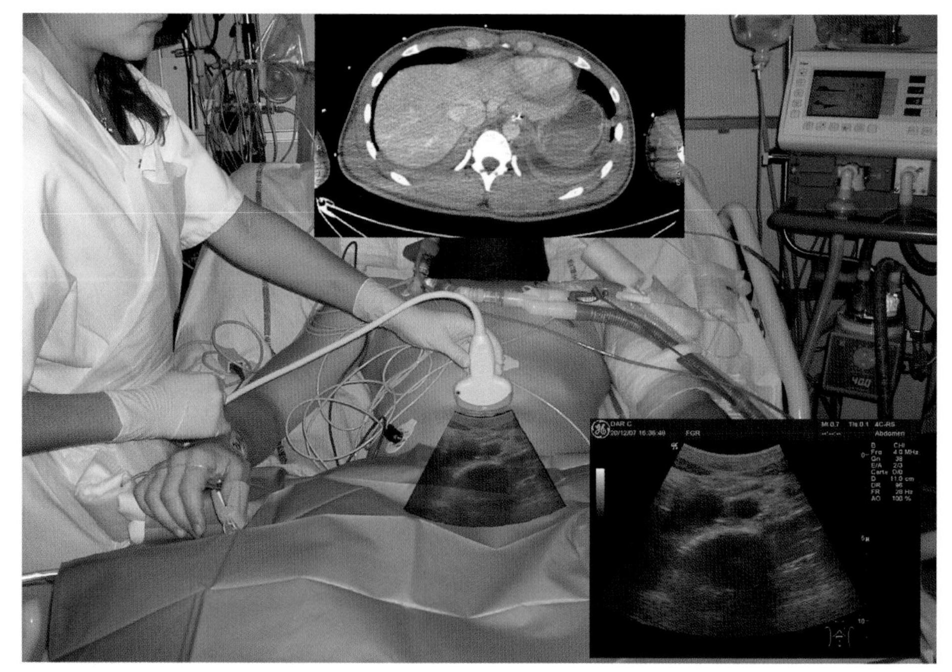

Transverse section

So that everyone concurs, it is agreed in general echography that, for the transverse section, the left of the screen represents the right of the patient and the right of the screen is the left of the patient. As is the case for the scanner! In longitudinal section, the left of the patient represents the patient's cephalic extremity (toward the head) and the right of the screen represents the patient's caudal extremity (toward feet).

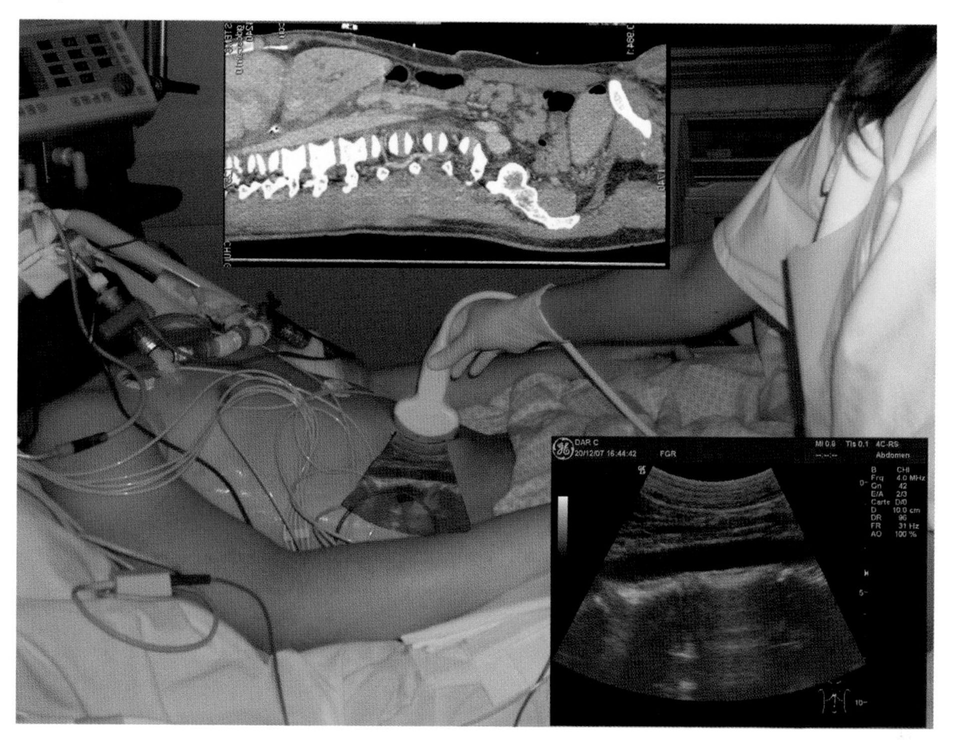

Longitudinal section

Thus, you just check the logo on the screen is indeed on the left, and you place the mark of the probe on the right side of the patient, or toward the head, according to the section you want. It is possible to do the contrary reversing the position of the mark on the screen (there is a switch for it), or reversing the position of the probe. In the end, the most important is to be able to find one's bearings. Moreover, this agreement is different for cardiologists, but that's another story.

Now that we are professionals of sections, we do a longitudinal section putting the probe on the axillary line, perpendicular to the skin (on a patient lying on his back, the probe must be parallel to the bed plane). This section separates the chest from the back of the patient. It is called a frontal section (frontal because it is parallel to the forehead). People who want to remember that it is a longitudinal section on the side, it is perfect. Thus, the left of the screen is always toward the head and the right of the screen toward the feet.

To finish, notice that we usually place ourselves on the patient's right to do the echography, as for the clinical examination. This is the reason why the probes are generally placed on the right of the apparatus.

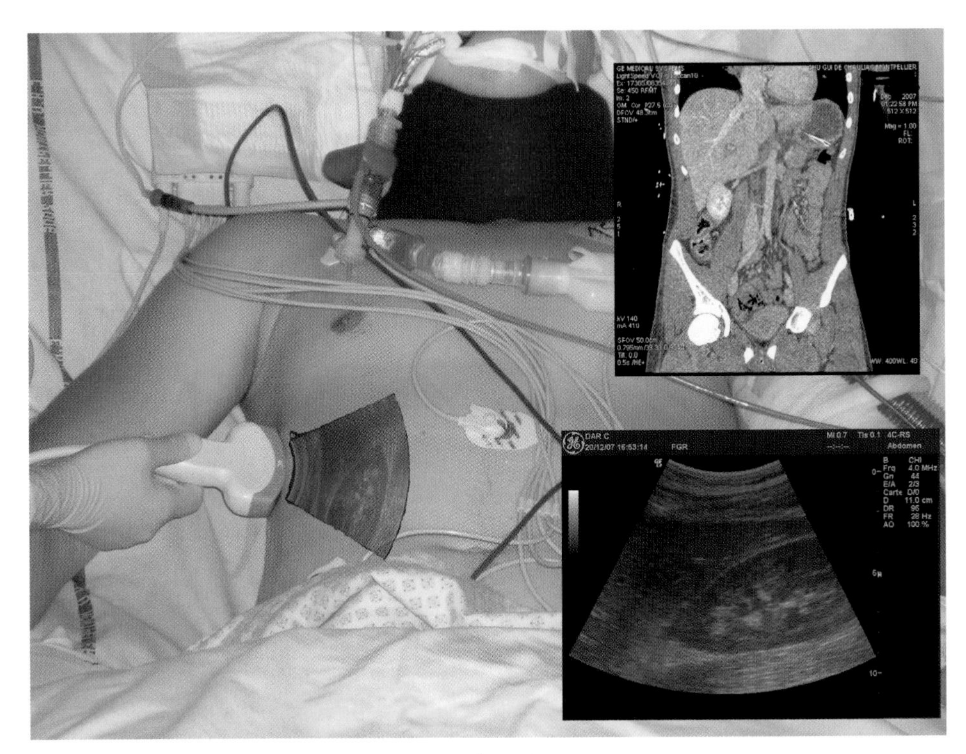

Frontal section

Here are the fruits of my labor, after so many nights observing the "creature."

■ The kidney, landmark of the abdomen

I came across a summary of a presentation made during the "Agora 2007," about training in emergency echography for neophytes. Puzzled, I contacted the author who rapidly explained to me the method.

"The essential in emergency medicine, face to a hypotensive patient, is to suppress as quickly as possible a surgical pathology, particularly in traumatology. The echography fully plays its part here. It is easy to implement, quick, it can be repeated and doesn't ray the patient and the staff."

The most important is to follow meticulously a program set in advance. This program describes a way along the chest and the abdomen of the patient, and permits to visualize the essential organs and answer the following questions: "Does the patient bleed within his thorax or abdomen? Does his heart beat normally? Is the heart compressed by blood or air? Is his abdominal aorta disrupted?"

To do so, let's start from the beginning. If the liver or spleen is damaged, it will start bleeding in the abdominal cavity and the blood will tend to gather in the space between the kidney and the liver (Morison's pouch), between the kidney and the spleen, and around the bladder (pouch of Douglas). Fresh blood is a liquid, thus anechogenic (black) in echography. So you have to search BLACK between the liver and the kidney, between the spleen and the kidney, and around the bladder.

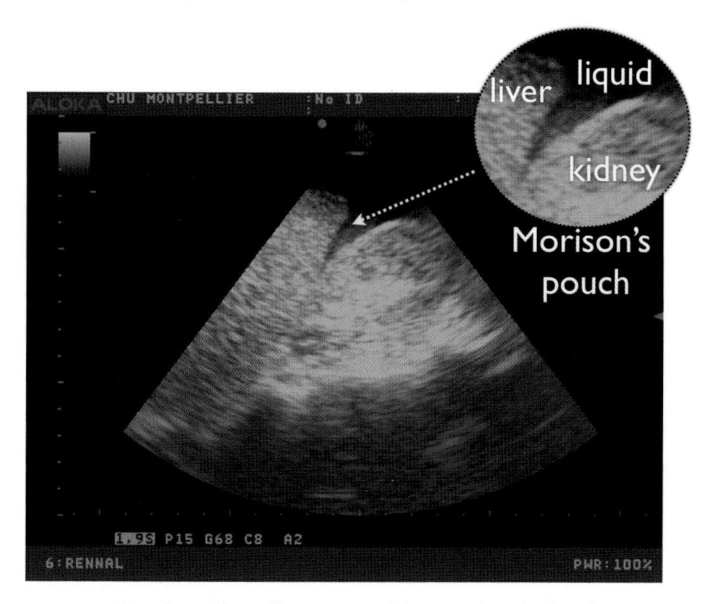

Road accident: liver wound, hemorrhagic shock

The steps

First step: find the right kidney. First, let's explore Morison's pouch. To find it, we will use the kidney as our target. The kidney is a bean-shaped organ composed of two parts: the cortex (peripheral), which is blood-filled and thus not very echogenic; and the medulla (central), composed of an entanglement of collecting ducts surrounded by connective tissues that are very echogenic. Finding the kidney is like hunting out a bean that is black all around and white in the center.

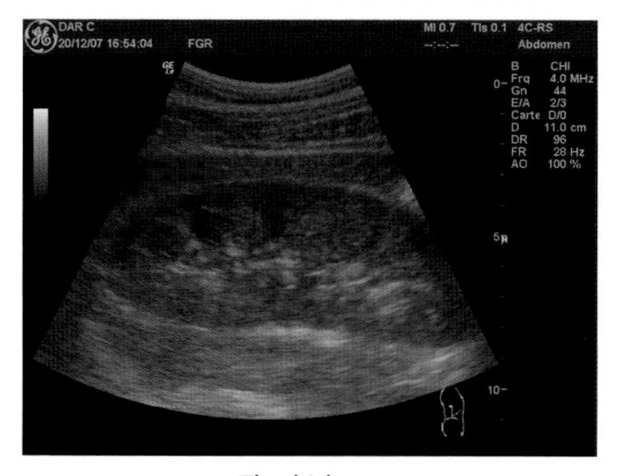

The kidney

The kidney is generally located more than 8 cm deep. Therefore we need to use a low-frequency probe, and, ideally, an abdominal probe.

We will consistently make longitudinal sections of the right side from the axillary pit toward the iliac bone, along the anterior axillary line, then along the medium axillary line, and finally the posterior one, until we find the kidney. For now, we should not take an interest in other visualized structures but only concentrate on the KIDNEY.

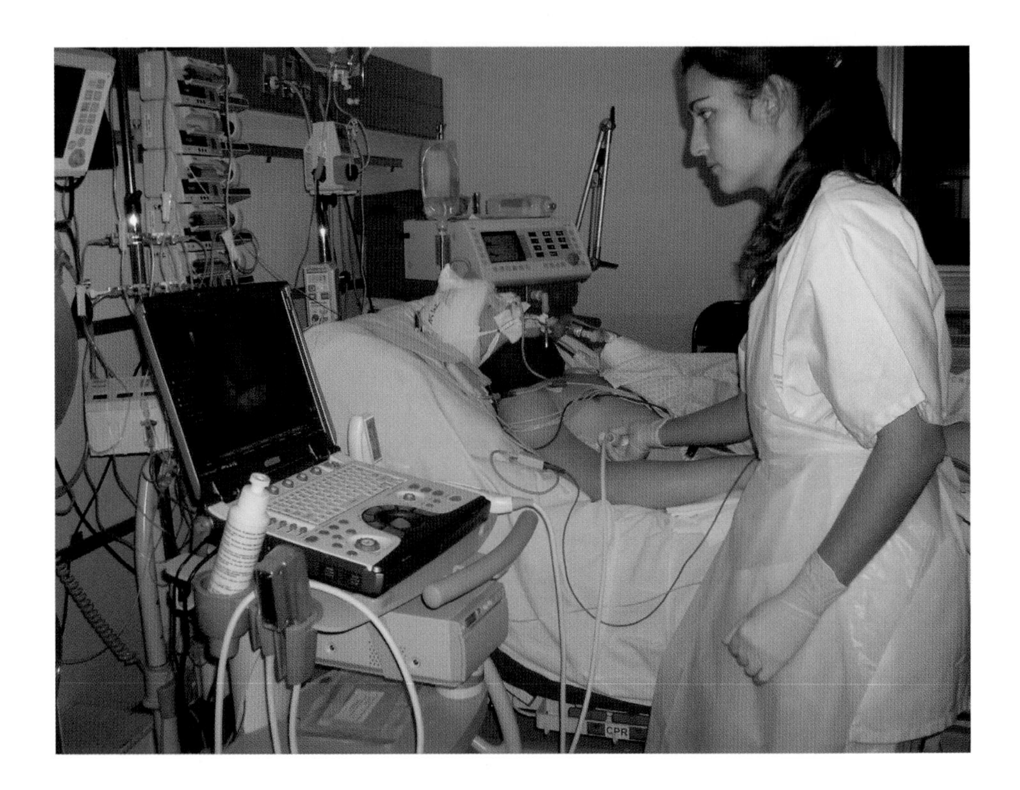

If, after the consistent exploration, the kidney isn't found out, do it again. If, in spite of a second exploration, you can't find the kidney, you should move on to the next stage before repeating the consistent exploration of the kidney. Inevitably, you will find the kidney (of course if the patient has his two kidneys!).

Once you have found the kidney, the structure that we can see above it (on the left of the screen) is the liver. Above the liver, the white line represents the diaphragm and above it, the lung. This is how we become specialists in anatomy.

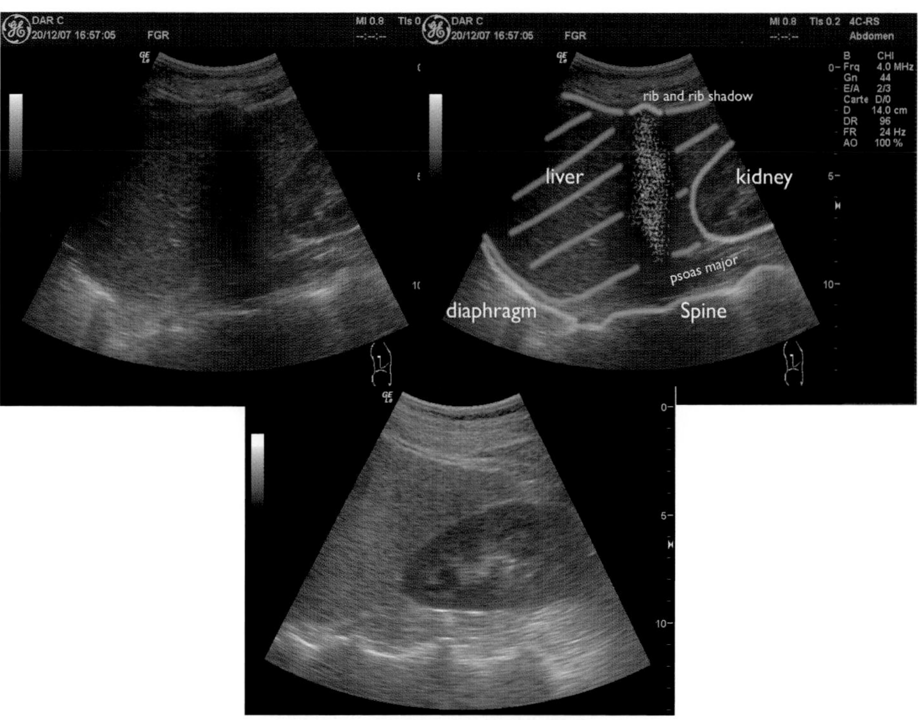

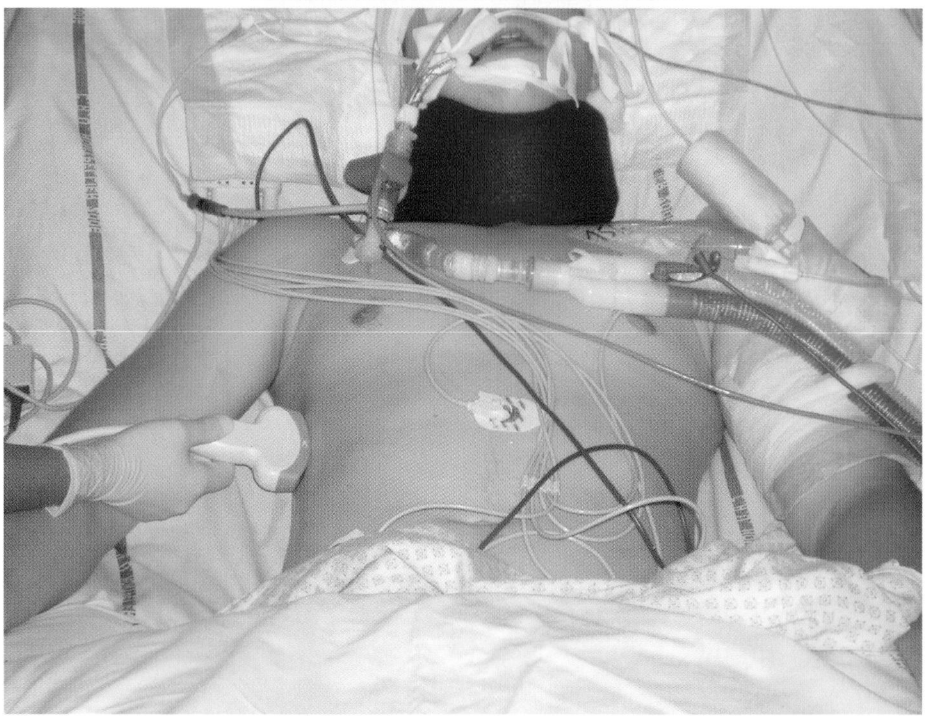

Morison's pouch between kidney and liver

The only question that remains is: *"Does some black separate the liver from the kidney?"*

Repeat this methodology until it becomes familiar. This consistent longitudinal movement of the probe up and down as if you are ploughing the area is called gridding.

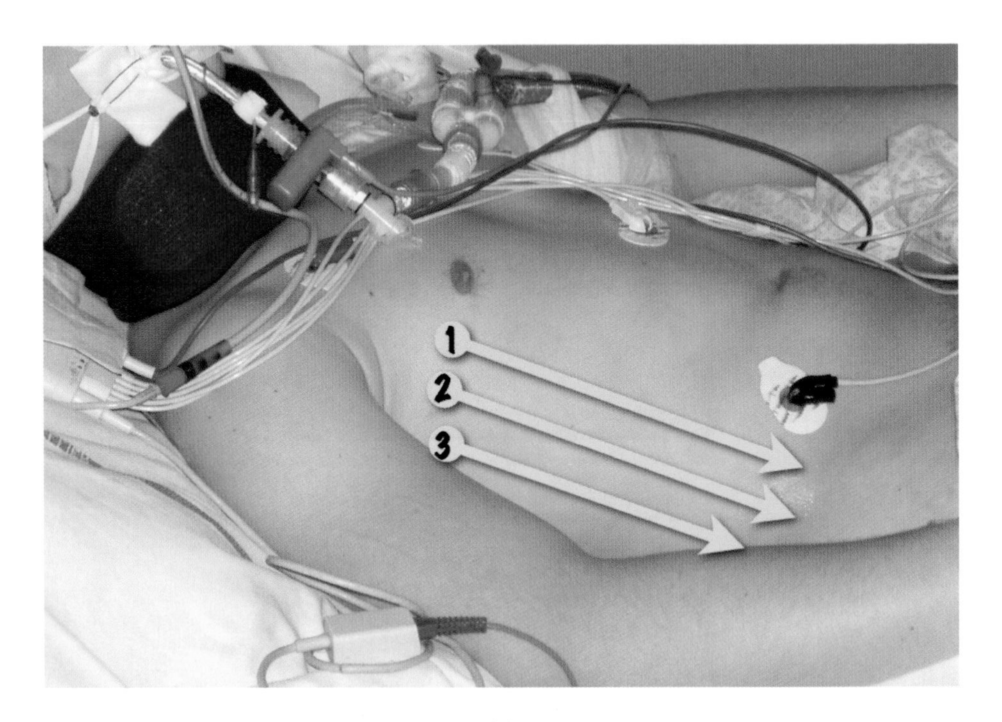

Gridding

Second step: Find the left kidney. Repeat exactly the same movements on the left side to search for the left kidney. The organ above it is the spleen. Remember that, generally speaking, you should not be afraid of gridding more in the future.

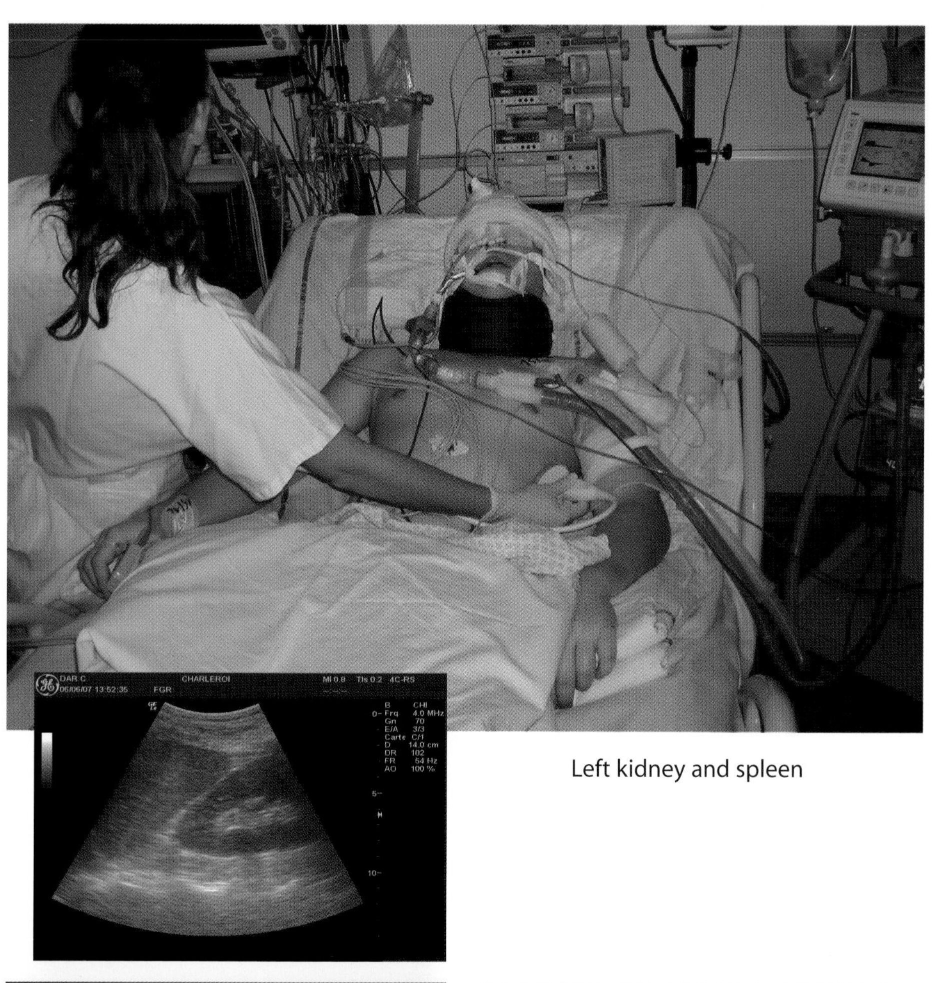

Left kidney and spleen

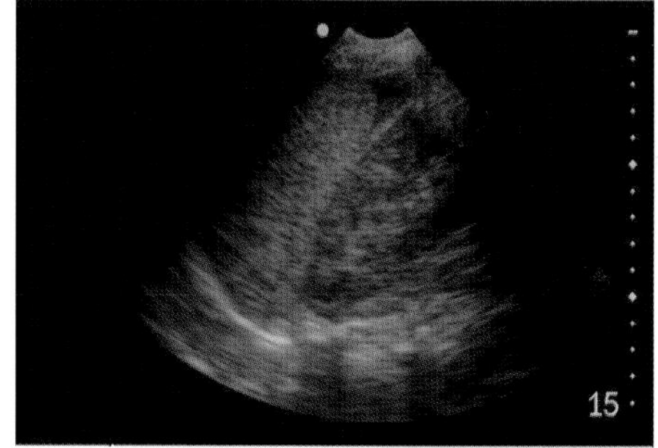

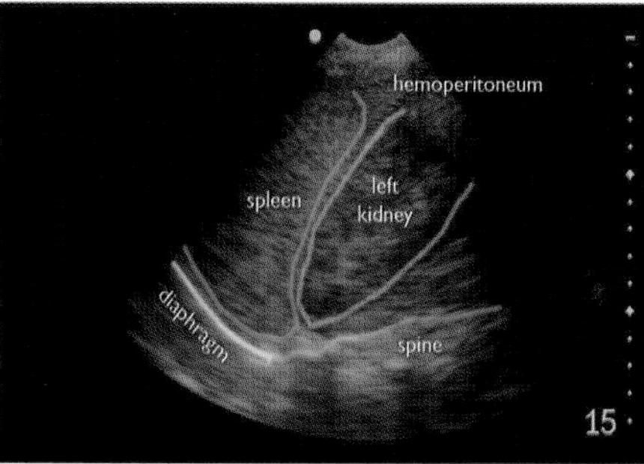

Horse accident: splenic contusion, moderate hemoperitoneum,
no hemodynamic instability, conservative treatment

Third step: Find the bladder. You should do a gridding on the midline, sliding the transducer from the umbilicus to the pubis. When you come up against the pubis, you have to lean the transducer toward the feet in order to see the pelvis. Normally, the bladder is visualized with a longitudinal section (black pouch with a white line around). The top of the bladder (on the left of the screen) is called the bladder dome, and you have to search for some black around and behind it. If you can't localize the bladder, either it is empty or you have slipped and are not anymore on the midline of the body.

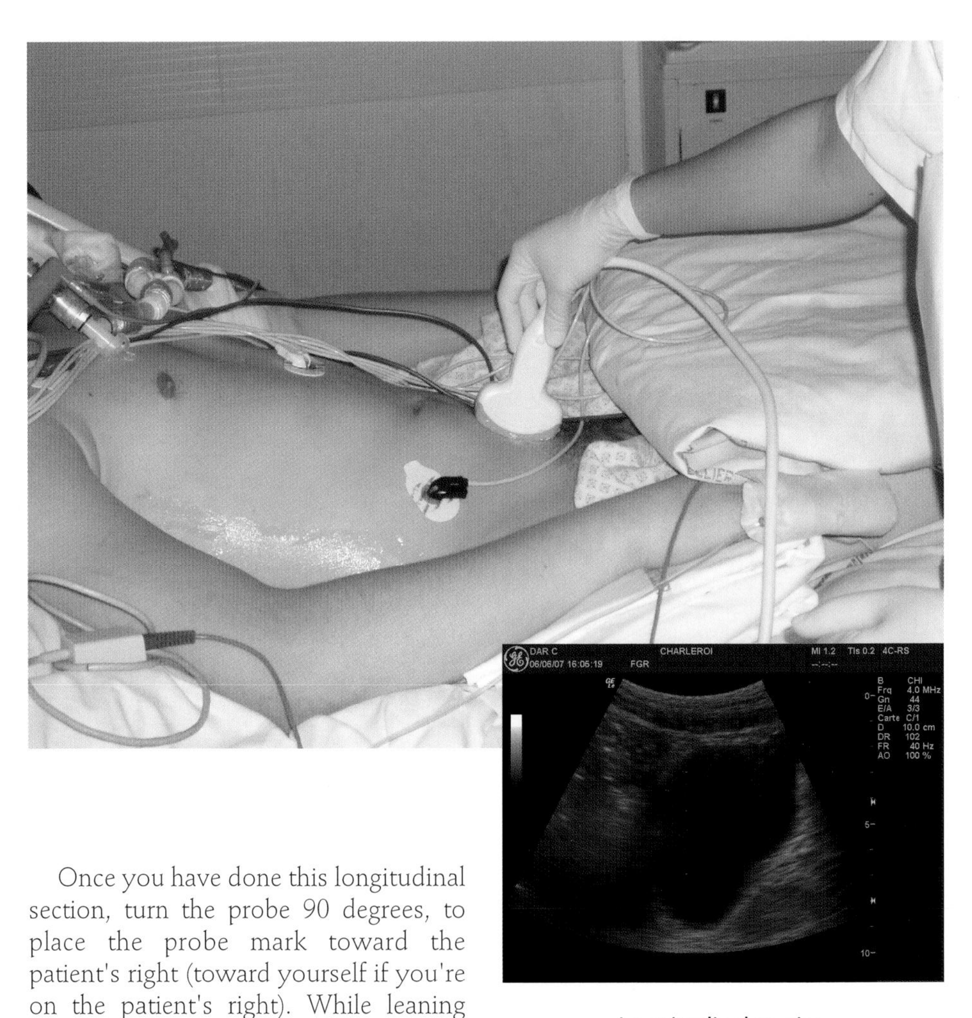

Longitudinal section of the bladder

Once you have done this longitudinal section, turn the probe 90 degrees, to place the probe mark toward the patient's right (toward yourself if you're on the patient's right). While leaning first toward the patient's feet and then toward his head, you will explore in transverse section the Douglas pouch to search for some black.

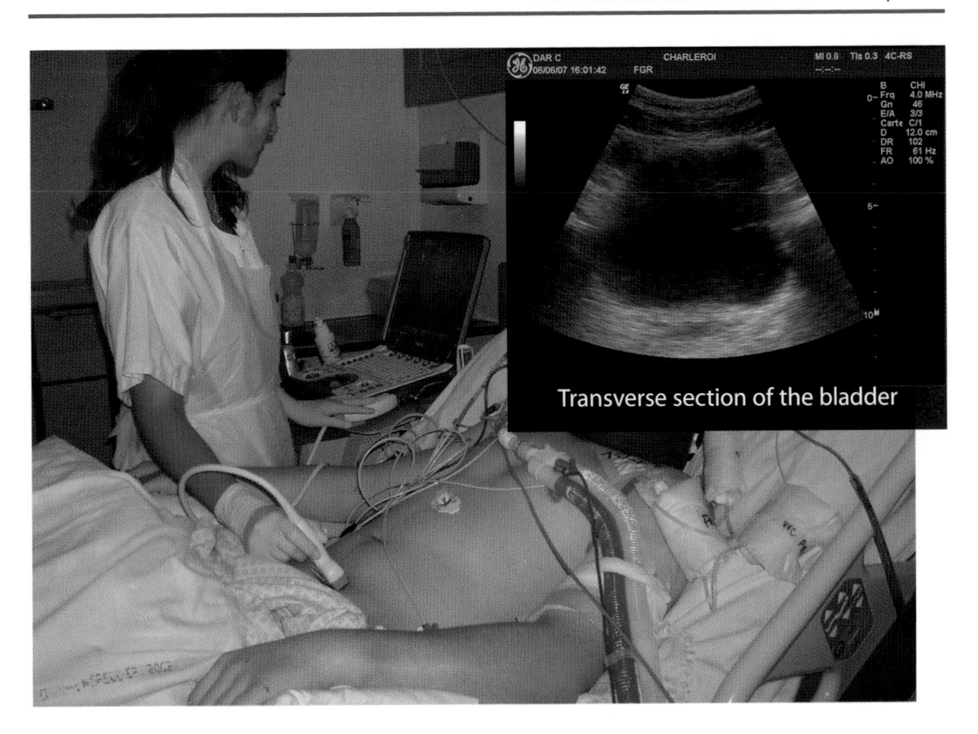

Transverse section of the bladder

These first three steps permit to assert or not the presence of liquid in the abdominal cavity, and even in the thoracic cavity because we have explored the pleural pouches when gridding from the axillary pit. If you had seen some black above the diaphragm, it would have answered our question. But that's another story.

Fourth step: Find the heart. You should keep the probe transversely and place it perpendicular to the skin in the epigastric fossa. On the screen, you must see two black rounds, the aorta on the right and the vena cava on the left of the screen. Both are located in front of the lumbar spine represented by a semicircular white line that creates a posterior shadow cone. When you push the probe, you can see that the vena cava disappears. If you can only see the aorta, relax the pressure of the probe and, as if by magic, you will see the vena cava. If you lean the transducer to look at the patient's head from under the ribs, following the vena cava, you will find a structure in motion. It is the heart. Set the inclination of the probe and the depth as well as possible. This subcostal view permits you to visualize the heart through the liver. The question is: "How does it beat?" and you have to search for a black space between the heart and the liver, which could correspond to a pericardial effusion.

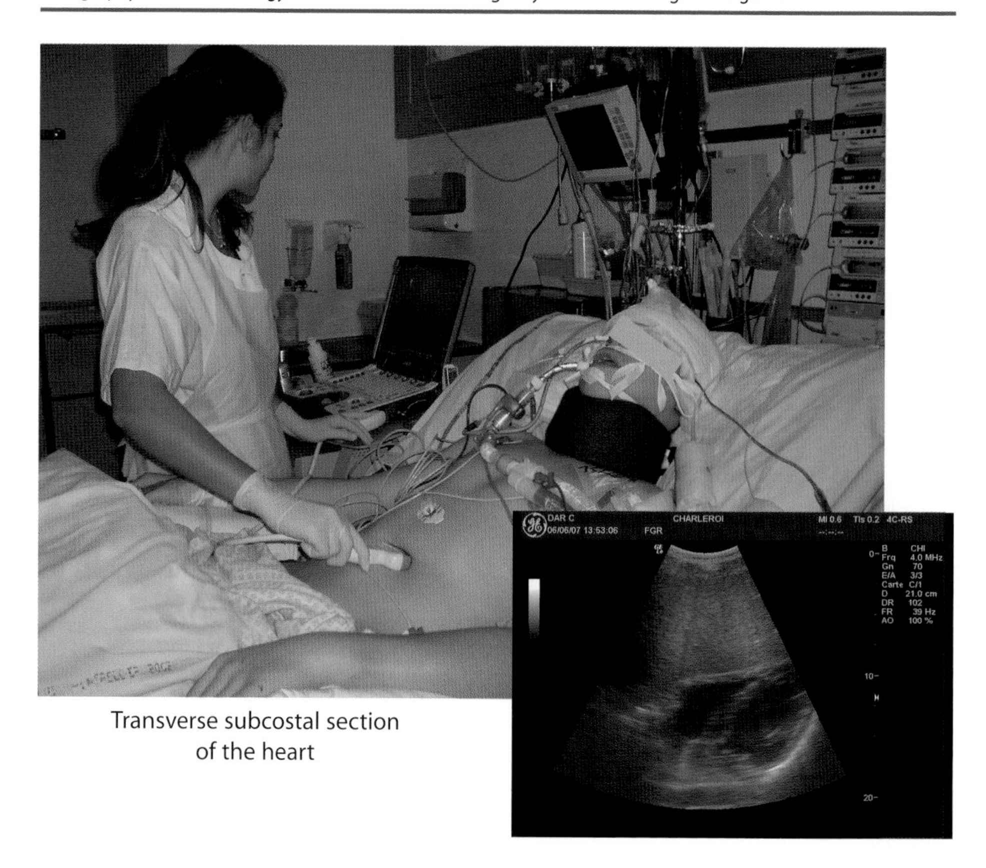

Transverse subcostal section of the heart

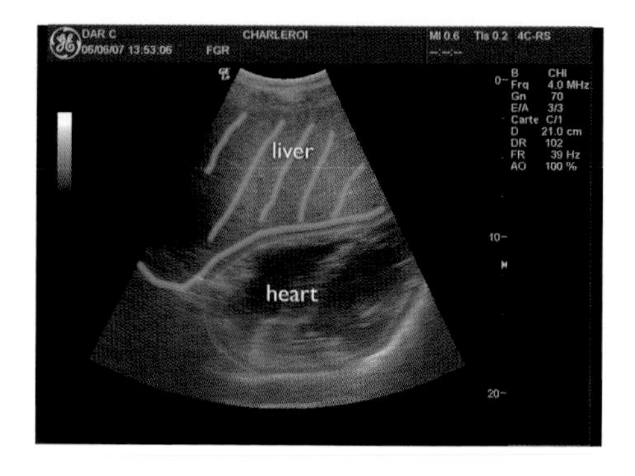

Fifth step: Find the aorta. It consists in lifting the probe and coming back to the visualization of the vena cava and aorta with a transverse section, sliding the transducer downwards, so that we can explore the abdominal aorta to search an abdominal aneurysm.

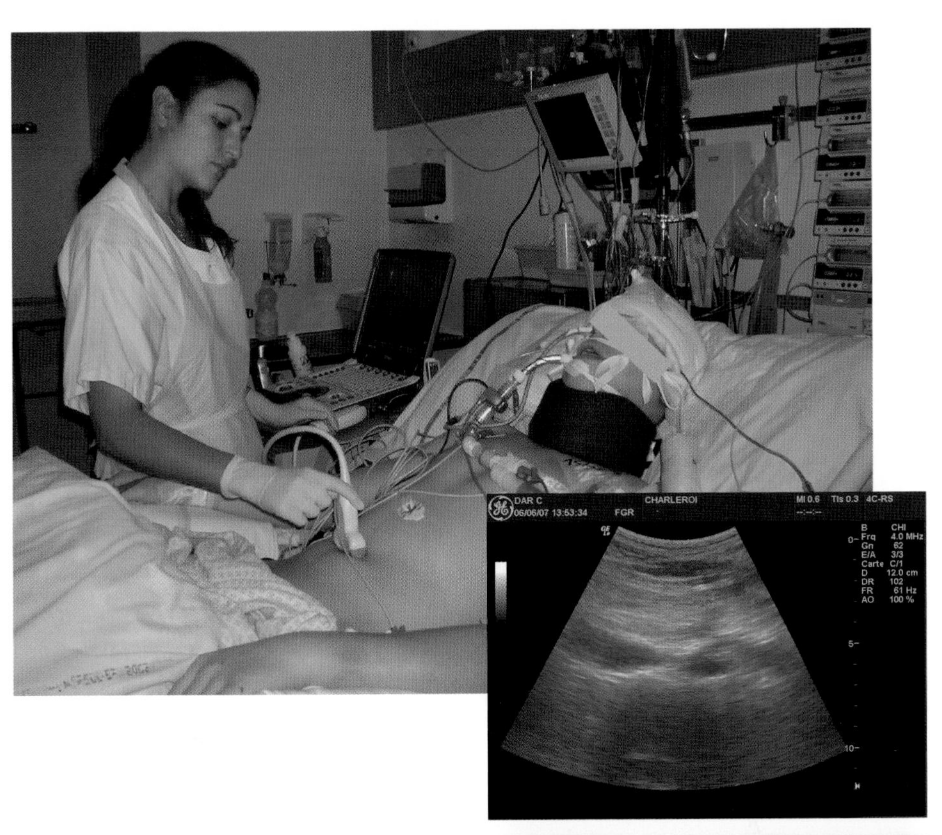

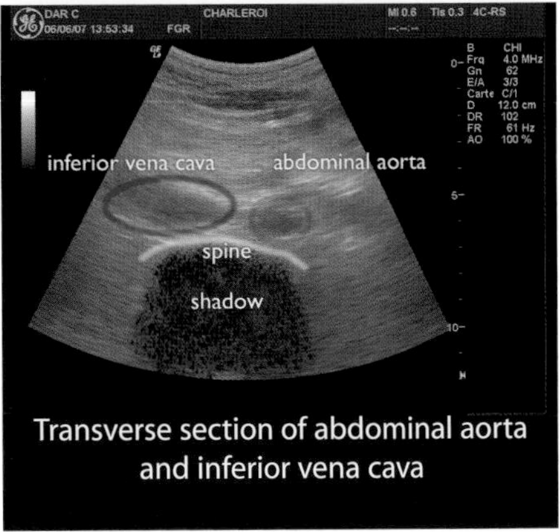

Transverse section of abdominal aorta and inferior vena cava

A longitudinal section will complete the examination of the aorta, searching for the loss of parallelism of the walls.

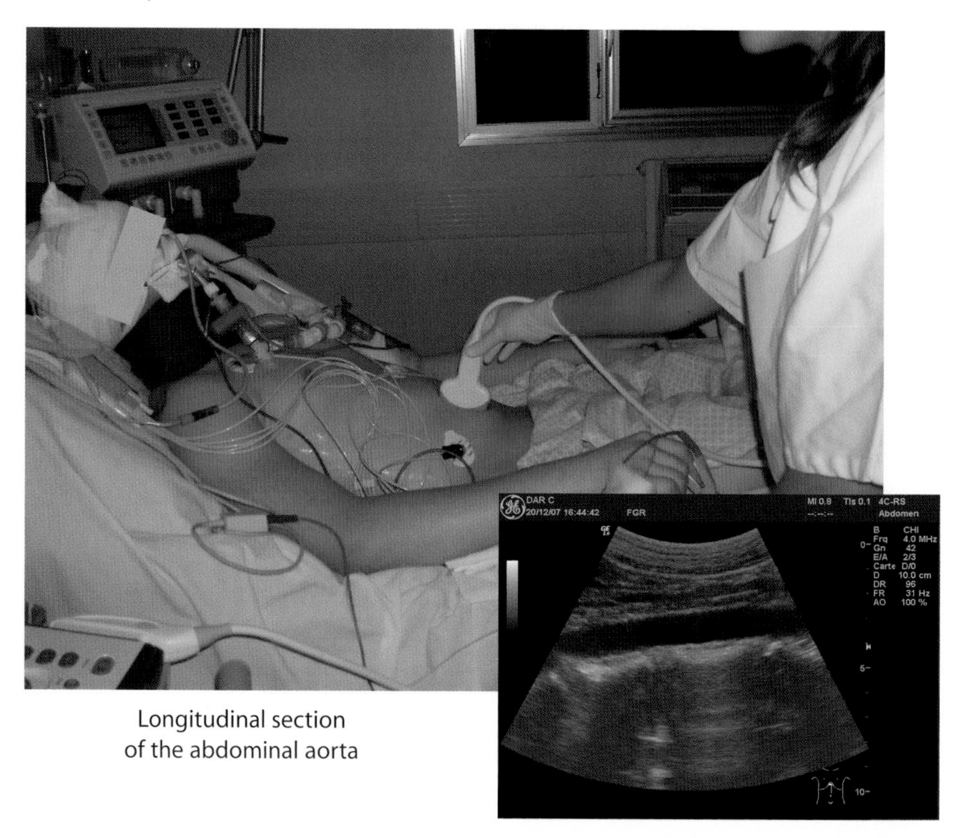

Longitudinal section of the abdominal aorta

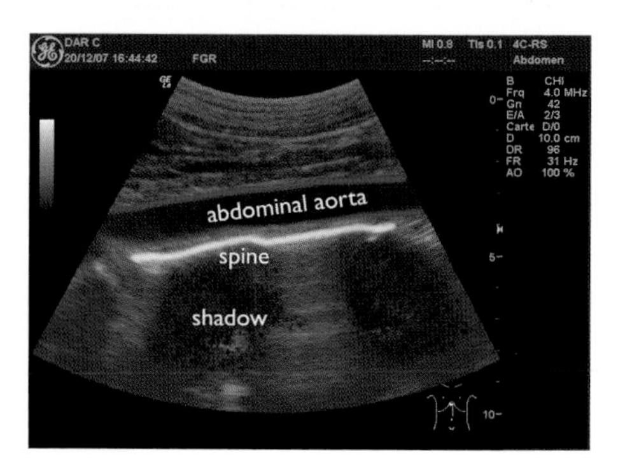

A diameter less than 25 millimeters will rule out the possibility of an anomaly of the abdominal aorta. To take the measure, there is on every machine a very similar procedure. Nevertheless, to do it faster, it is possible to compare the diameter to the depth scale displayed on the right of the screen. It is inaccurate, but it can be useful for a person who doesn't know the machine.

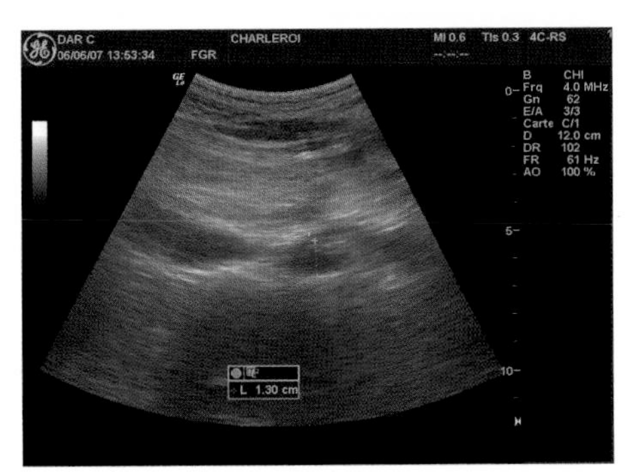

Measuring the anteroposterior diameter of the abdominal aorta

Here is, briefly, the crash program. In order to be efficient in the emergency department, you should repeat it tirelessly so that you acquire the gesture, first with a healthy patient. After 2 hours of training, the beginner will be able to perform the program in 3 minutes, and soon, with a little experience, in 40 seconds. Turning on the echograph is what takes most time.

I recommend you, then, to do the course again, a book in the hand, and to try and better understand the structures you visualize. Feel free to take this walk with your radiologist colleague.

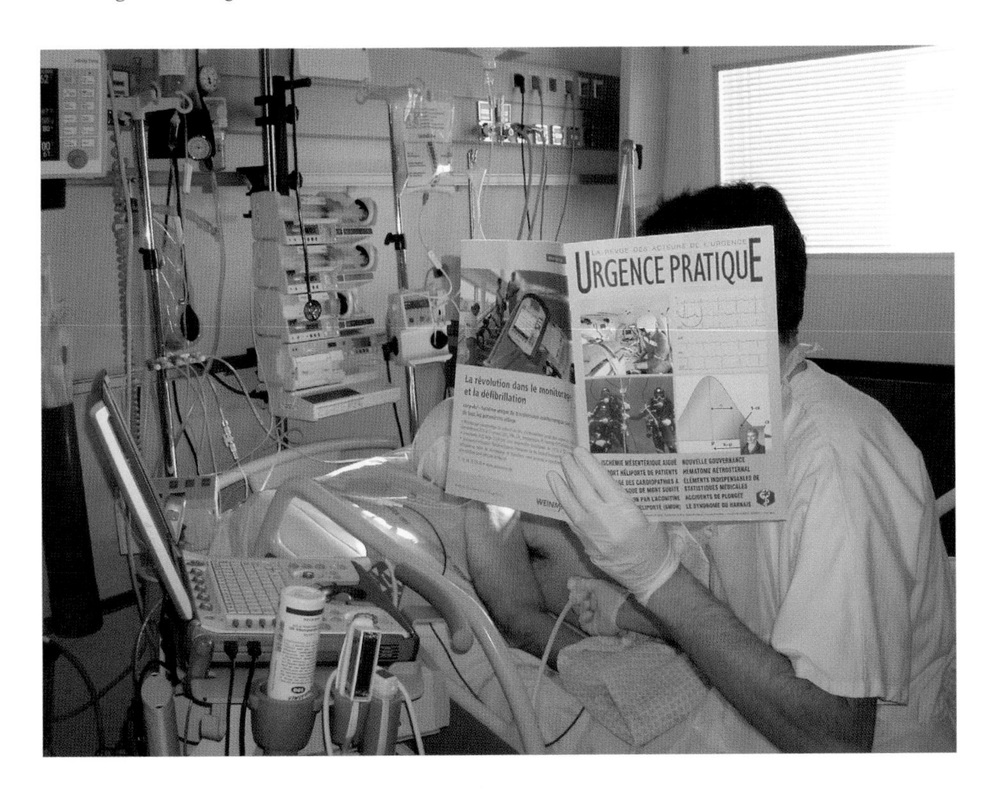

As I was rather disbelieving, I shut myself away in a room of intensive care, with an intubated and ventilated patient, and tested the training method. I applied it without thinking, concentrating myself upon methodology.

I was very surprised to master it in less time than I thought. I came back the following nights, with the echography book I had borrowed from the radiologist, and tried to perfect my initiation. Some days later, I had to release the patient and start in the real world of emergency.

The doctor, the machine, and the patient in front of the screen

(So, we are draining?)

■ What a lot of water!

While I was on duty, as every night, I was called by my colleague of emergency department for a young 26-year-old woman who, although she had spent several days sunbathing on the ice field with her survival suit, was pale and hypotensive. My colleague stated that the medical history had revealed diffuse abdominal pain with guarding located in the lower abdomen on the right, intrauterine device (IUD), late period, a right annexial mass, and blood during the gynecological examination. As the diagnosis wasn't particularly mysterious, he confirmed me that the pregnancy test was positive and the β-HCG was being analyzed. Last detail, hemoglobin was at 9.99 g/dL. The surgeon was on the road back. He thanked me for letting him go to sleep. When the simple intensive care measures were taken, I took advantage of the situation to confirm our feeling and switched the machine on. The echographic examination found without any doubt BLACK between the liver and the kidney and around the bladder. As for the uterus, it presented echoes in itself where we seem to distinguish a sort of stem that could be the IUD but I saw nothing more familiar. The whole image confirmed the presence of an intra-abdominal effusion that, in this context, referred to a hemoperitoneum.

The surgical operation confirmed the diagnosis of extra-uterine pregnancy.

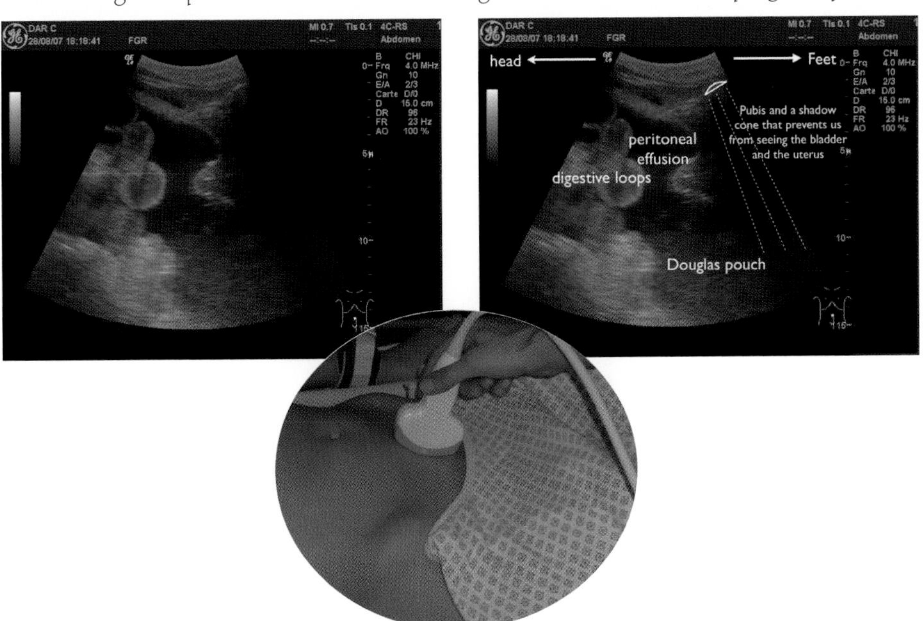

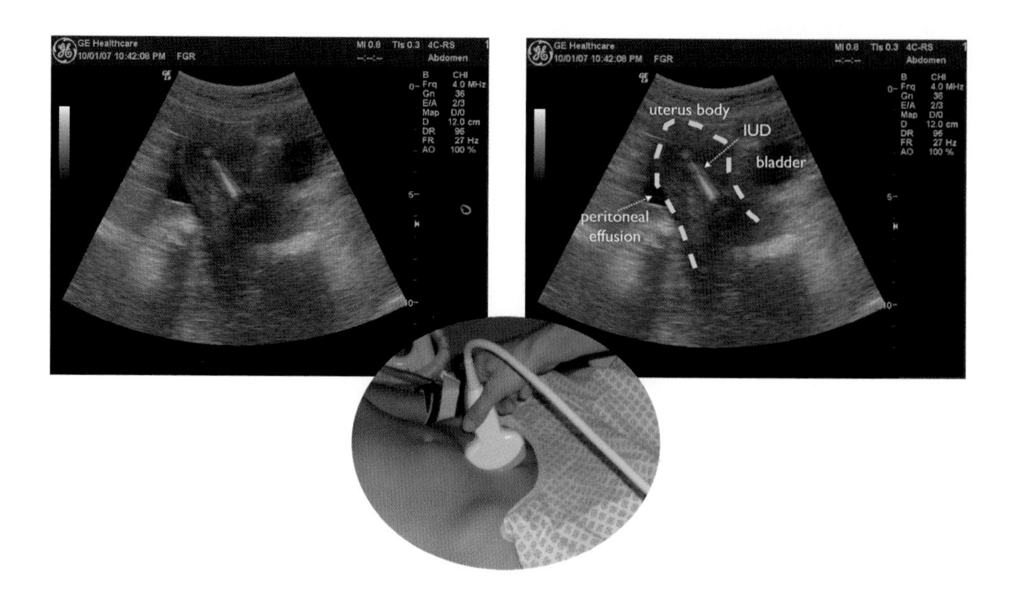

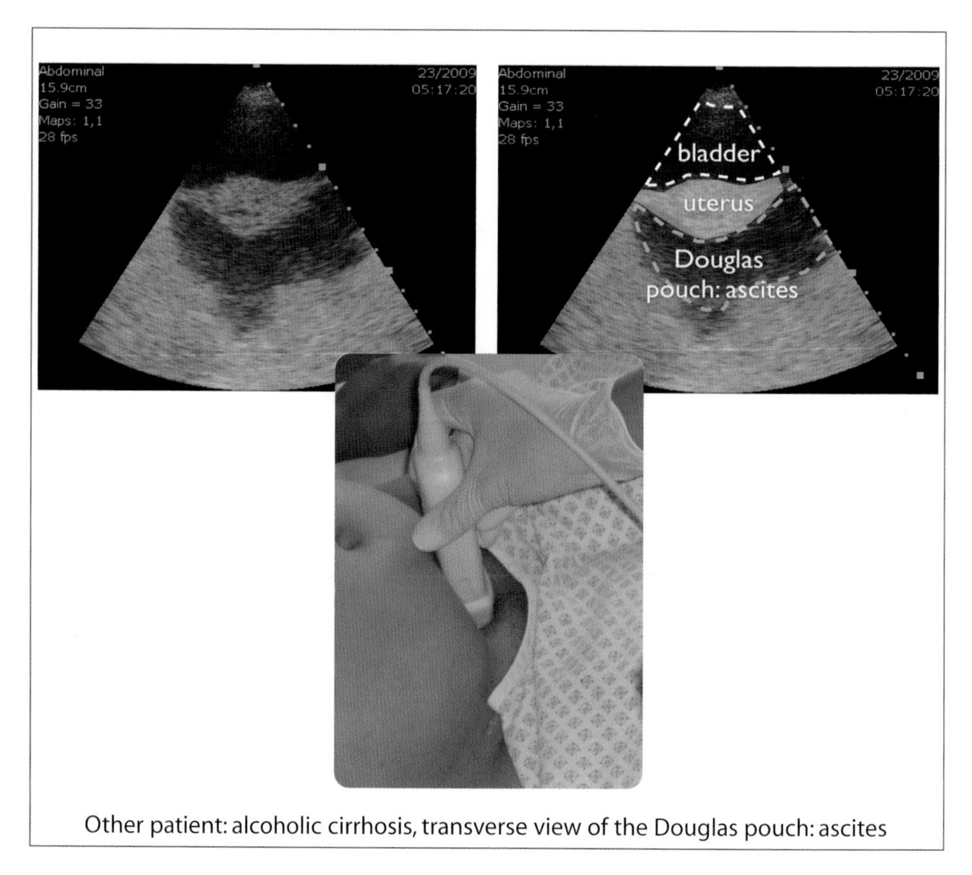

Other patient: alcoholic cirrhosis, transverse view of the Douglas pouch: ascites

■ In a fix

As he was going to work (what was he going to do in such a drag?), in the early morning, a 29-year-old man crashed his snowmobile into a tree that had just sprouted during the night. He was taken into charge and immediately brought to the emergency department where we laid him down on a stretcher. His examination through clothes revealed that we had to undress him to see more. The aware patient complained about a pain in the thorax and in the right leg. The checkup revealed a closed fracture of the right tibia and a fracture of the sternum. I took the opportunity to practice and moved the probe around without seeing anomalies. Morison, Douglas, and Sir Pericardium were dry.

We took the patient to the operation room and operated his leg under combined blocks with a propofol sedation.

Two days later, I was called to orthopedics. The nurse, with good reason, was worried because the patient was agitated, dyspneic, pale, hypotensive, and in a sweat. The patient said he didn't feel right, his chest hurt, and he had a feeling of imminent death. The pulse was not easily perceptible; it was quick and thread, varying with the breathing movements, reminding of a paradoxical pulse. The jugular veins were turgescent, the pulmonary examination was symmetric, and the heart sounds were remote. The patient under oxygen and with an adapted filling was immediately taken to the recovery room. Face to this clinical situation, evoking a tamponade, we used the echographic machine while waiting for the thorax radiography. The pleura and the peritoneum were dry. As for the heart, it floated over a "pericardial pool." It struggled to ensure his owner's survival. Seeing the emergency of the situation, we opened a central line equipment and, thanks to a transverse subcostal view, an echographic location permitted to have an idea of the shortest way (location, direction, and depth of the puncture) to find oil. Some antiseptic solution, a drape, gloves, and the needle mounted on a syringe followed the direction shown previously by the probe.

When the needle reached the calculated depth, a blood reflux without pulse and an immediate improvement were the sign of the mission's success. We disconnected the syringe, brought forward the metallic guide, and, glancing at the ECG, removed the syringe. After a cutaneous dilatation, we placed the central venous catheter in the pericardium and removed the guide. Altogether, 550 milliliters of bloody liquid was removed to the patient's great relief. Since there was no recurrence, we removed the drain 48 hours later. We found no other etiology except the initial thorax trauma. And of course, the preventive anticoagulant agent was just right to be guilty!

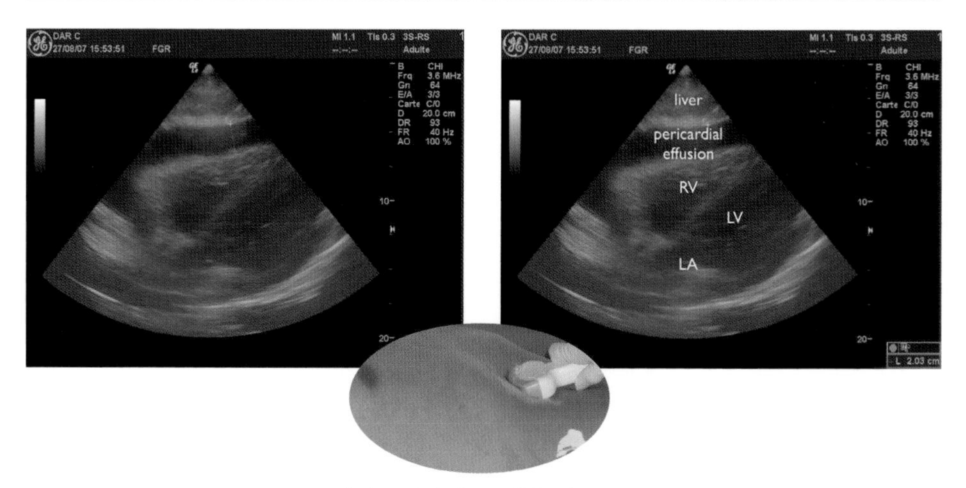

Subcostal view of the heart

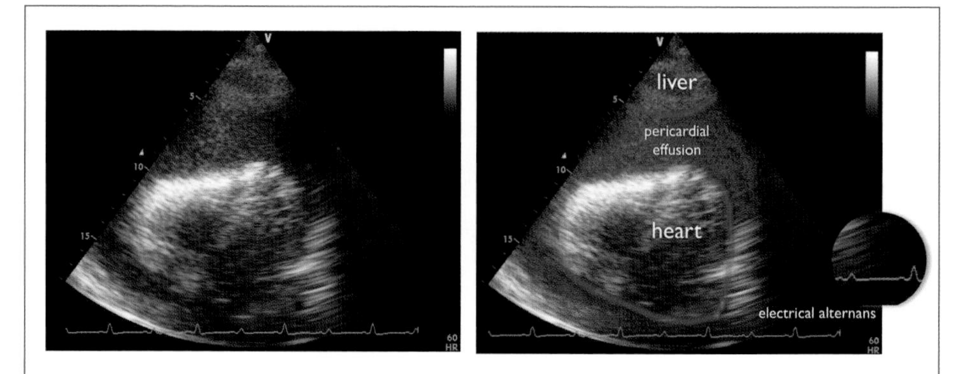

Other patient: progressively appearing dyspnea, tachycardia, distended jugular veins, electrical alternans: neoplastic pericardial effusion

A little suds?

I'd been called in Cardiology Intensive Care Department for a patient with respiratory insufficiency with fever. Wondering why the patient was hospitalized in cardiology while he seemed to suffer from a pneumonitis, I quickly understood, thanks to the medical staff's distraught expression, that things were going bad. A quick look at the patient's blue lips dotted with foam started me thinking. Without a word, the unconscious patient was intubated and ventilated. A lot of foam went out by the intubation probe. Ventilation with 100% of oxygen with PEEP and a few amines and furosemide permitted the patient to get his color back. As for myself, I had become as white as the staff. The clinical examination found crepitations on both pulmonary fields; the heartbeat sounds were quick and regular, with a gallop noise but no obvious murmur. We didn't notice any edema in inferior limbs. On the contrary, we saw a hepatojugular reflux. The ECG showed a diffuse elevation without Q waves and the troponin, sampled a few hours earlier, was high. I turned on the echographic machine, and a consistent exploration permitted to see a big heart with a subcostal transverse section, a big heart that didn't seem to contract that much: in short, a hypokinetic heart. With this fever, all these clues evoked an infectious myocarditis, confirmed by the cardiologist.

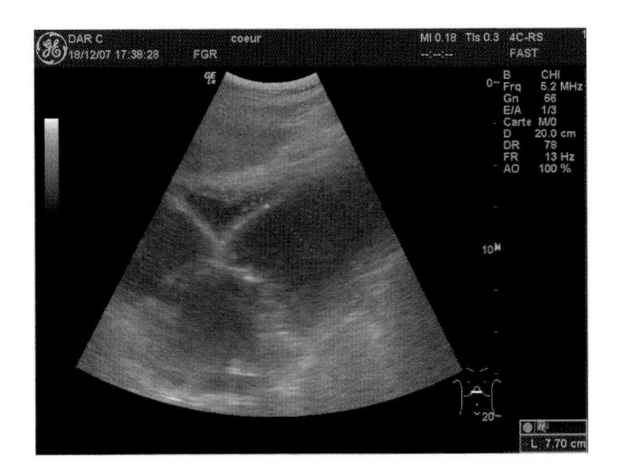

Subcostal view: dilatation of the left ventricle and atria. The right ventricle cannot be well seen (hypokinesia is obvious in dynamic view).

The systolic function of the left ventricle is easily estimated, thanks to the only vision of the beating heart. In most cases, a subcostal transverse section permits to see the heart, particularly with an intubated and ventilated patient, using the liver as an echographic window. During a cardiac arrest, the absence of any cardiac activity is a sign of poor prognosis that suppresses any chance to recover a cardiac activity. If the subcostal view can't be used (bandage or failure), don't hesitate to grid the thorax looking for something moving.

■ Don't push!

"NO, you won't keep me here any longer, I want to go back home." "But don't even think of it, sir, you have to fill in the urinal." Woken up by this verbal exchange, usual in the waiting room of outpatient surgery, I quickly understood that Mr. Diesel, living face to the hospital, on the other side of the snow heap, and who was operated for hemorrhoids this morning under spinal anesthesia, wanted to go back home. Fortunately, the protocol was against him: no urine, no home! As I wished to resume my nap and also knew the quick temper of both protagonists, I turned on the echographic machine to estimate the bladder volume.

In transverse section, I measured the bladder width and its depth, while its length in centimeters was measured in longitudinal section on the midline. I multiplied these three measures by each other and divided the total by 2. This resulted in a volume of 100 milliliters. We could understand, with so little urine in his bladder, why Mr. Diesel wasn't that much fine.

As he had no sign of urinary retention, the patient, so proud of having thumbed his nose at the protocol, went home with the advice of coming back if he had any persistent dysuria. We didn't see him again.

We consider the bladder is very much like an ellipsoidal volume. I remind you that an ellipsoid, in mathematics, is a second-degree surface of the three-dimensional Euclidean space. Thus it is a type of quadric, with a main feature: it has no point at infinity. In short, it's a rugby ball.

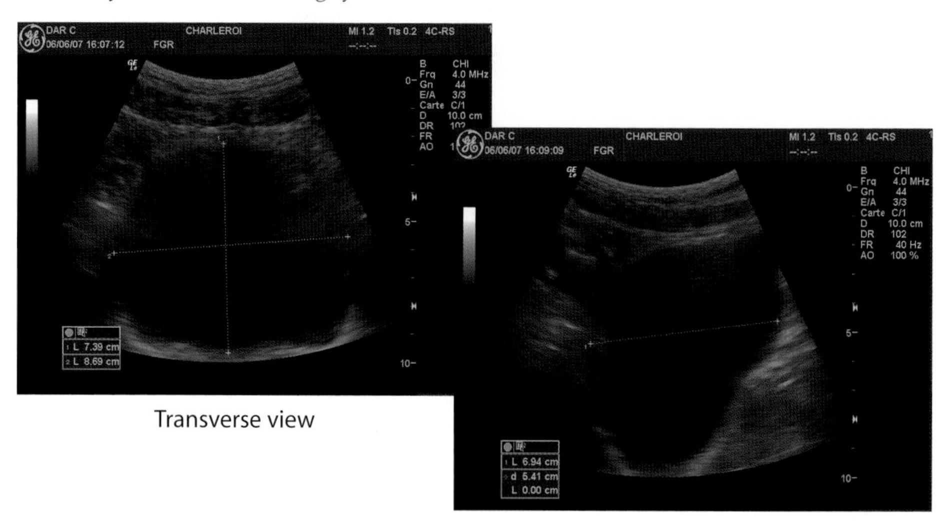

Transverse view

Longitudinal view of the bladder

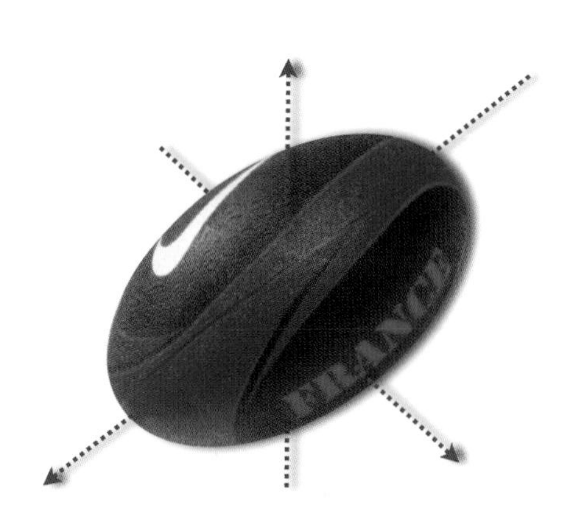

The volume of an ellipsoid is:
$4/3\pi abc$
where a, b, and c are strictly positive data, equal to the lengths of semi-axes of the object. As it is easier for us to measure ABC diameters than the radius, the equation becomes $\pi/3*(A*B*C)/2$ if we consider that π is almost equal to 3. The simplified equation results in an ellipsoid volume very near to $(A*B*C)/2$.

Longitudinal and transverse sections permit to obtain ABC in centimeters, and thus the volume in milliliters of the bladder.

The proof!

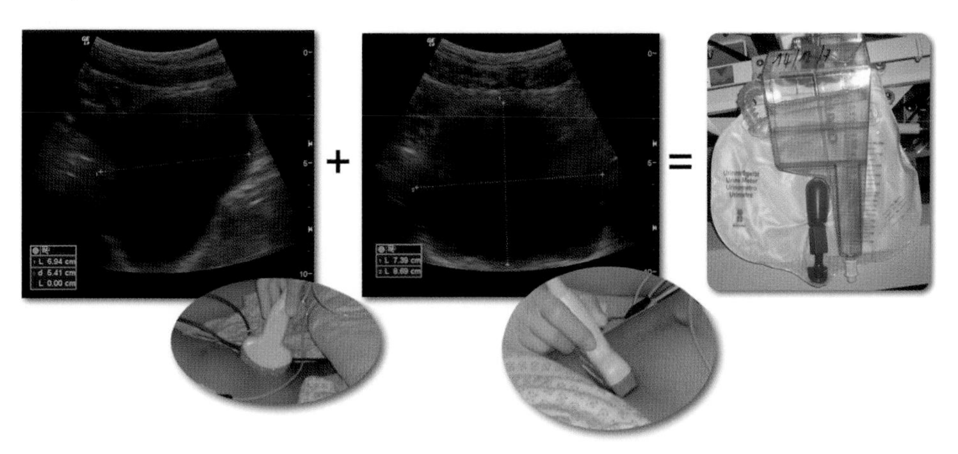

■ Out of breath

In postoperative from a surgery of the right hand under supraclavicular block, a 35-year-old man, professional trumpet player, complained he was short of breath. The patient was conscious. His respiratory frequency was 20 per minute; his blood pressure was 125/70 mmHg, and the oxygen saturation was 99% on room air. The thoracic inspection showed a less mobile hemithorax, and the auscultation revealed an asymmetry. The operating room FM radio seemed to resound more in the right side when the patient opened his mouth. The surgical bandage was clean and only a few blood drops were collected by the drain. In short, it was difficult to blame the surgeon.

As I suspected a pneumothorax, and the radiologist was busy setting his colleague's radio, I took the echograph. With the high-frequency probe, I could only establish that there was no sign of sliding without B line: confirmation of the diagnosis. The thorax radiography permitted to visualize a small pneumothorax, which was cured, thanks to a conservative treatment.

The pneumothorax diagnosis can be difficult for the beginner. The pulmonary echography is based on using artifacts because a normal lung, filled with air, cannot be seen. Air makes a perfect mirror for ultrasounds, strongly reflects sound waves, and thus produces a strong back current toward the transducer; then ultrasounds make several round trips between the probe and the air mirror, resulting in reverberation artifacts, which explain why the image is totally white. Indeed, although ultrasounds don't go beyond the pulmonary surface, their bouncing extends the time spent between their emission from the probe and their reception by the probe. The echograph thus concludes that the ultrasounds come from further, and creates these white echoes in depth. The pulmonary surface is made of the pleural line, which is very visible between two ribs. Echoes of reverberation will create this line again and again, at many different depths of the distance between the probe and the pulmonary surface (meaning I have bounced one, two, three times...).

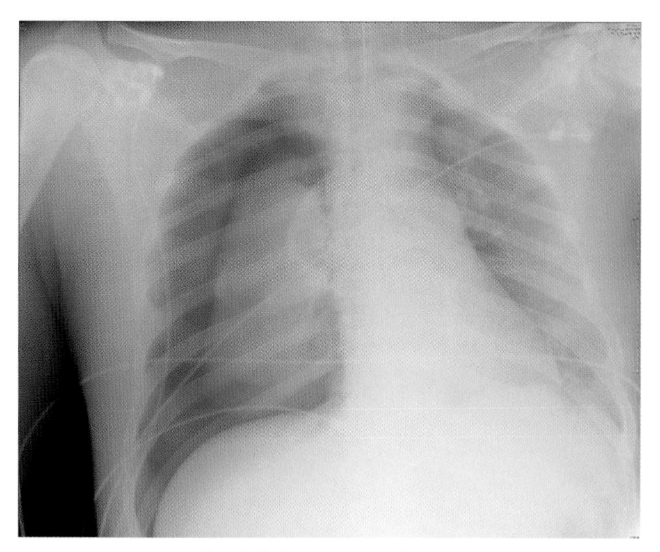

Total right pneumothorax

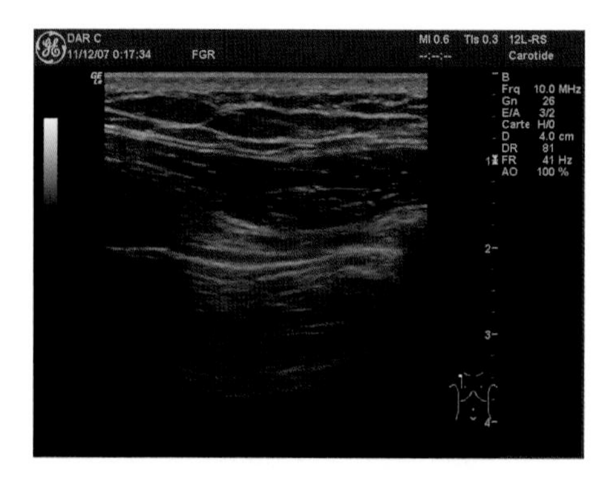

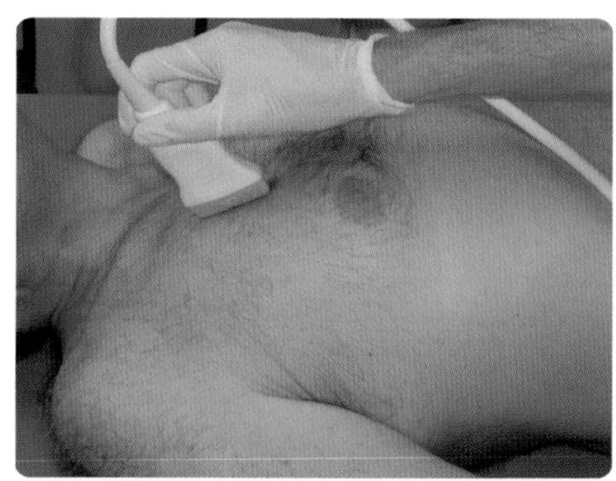

Immobile pleural line and no B line

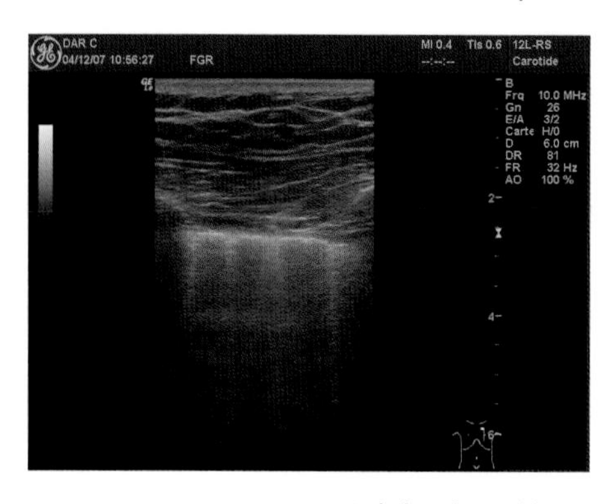

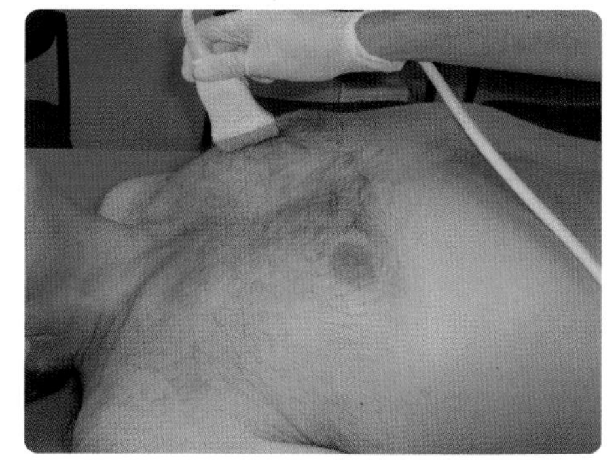

Mobile pleural line and presence of B lines

When we look at the pleural line, we can see that it is mobile and animated by a faint sizzling noise. Black points move within it at the rhythm of respiratory movements. This constitutes the pleural sliding, which is the visualization of the visceral pleura movement against the parietal pleura. In case of pneumothorax, there is air between the two pleurae. Yet, because of the air interposition, we can't see the visceral pleura anymore. As a consequence, there is no more pleural sliding.

B lines or "rockets" or "comet tails" are a feature of the pulmonary visceral pleura. They are dynamic phenomena, real ultrasound artifacts made of ephemeral longitudinal lines that go from the pleural line and go on without a break toward the lower part of the screen. Seeing them is seeing the lung, which eliminates any interposition of air between the two pleurae under the ultrasound beam.

To eliminate a pneumothorax, we should explore the whole thoracic wall. The echograph is preferably used to angle toward a positive diagnosis or eliminate a total pneumothorax, responsible for a tamponade symptomatology.

This is just the beginning to make your mouth water or to make your wall have some fresh air!

■ Charge!

A 40-year-old woman was brought to the emergency department by her husband, because of a strong pain in the left lumbar with urgent urination. The patient couldn't find a comfortable position. The pain had begun during the meal. First in the thorax, the patient said she would die because of this pain. Eventually, the pain was in the left lumbar region. Insensitive to paracetamol and ketoprofen administration, the patient was well soothed with morphine. The examination revealed a heart rate of 90 per minute, a blood pressure of 155/75 mmHg, and a temperature of 37,8°C (100°F). The cardiopulmonary examination had no special feature: all the pulses were present, the belly was tender and sensitive in its whole, and we couldn't palpate any mass. The left renal percussion was painful, and the patient's urine was hematuric. The ECG had no special feature. Waiting for the basic radiological examinations to be done, I took the opportunity to train. On the way, I didn't see anything particular but was surprised to find an abdominal aorta of normal size. Nevertheless, there was a hyperechogenic, mobile, linear image, which divided the aorta into two in its middle. Incredulous, I tried to set the machine better, thinking of an artifact; but whether in longitudinal or transverse section, the image was there. In the clinical context, it corresponded to an aortic dissection, which was confirmed by the scanner, and it even reached the left renal artery!

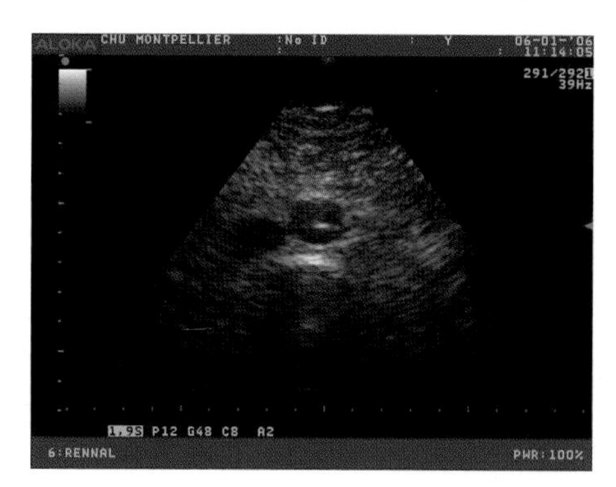

Transverse supra-umbilical section: inferior vena cava and abdominal aorta

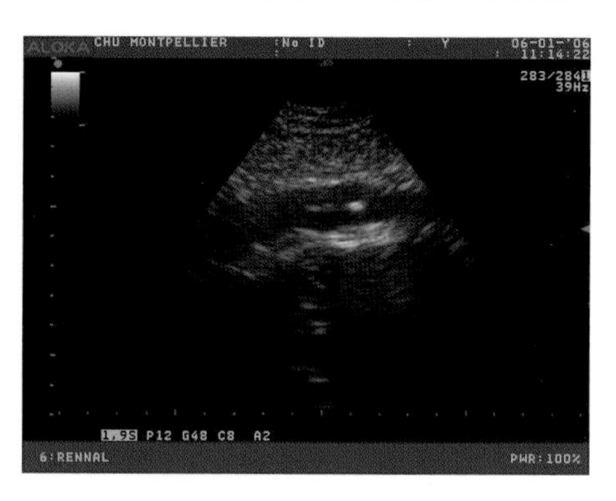

Longitudinal median supra-umbilical section: abdominal aorta

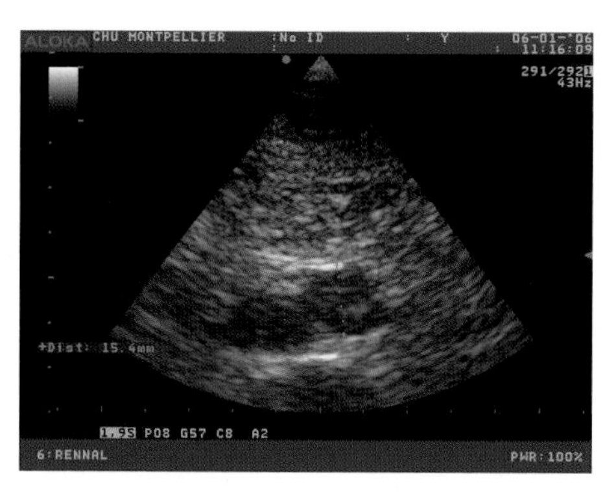

Transverse supra-umbilical section: no aortic dilatation but presence of a dissection

The diagnosis of abdominal aortic dissection is easy, but we have to think of it. To do so, we must not only look at the aorta and measure it but we particularly have to look for an unattached element within it. Thus it is logical to go and see the heart. Sometimes we are surprised to find a first image of the left ventricle that is hard to interpret for neophytes: it is the dilated aorta.

■ Take cover, it's going to explode!

A 60-year-old man, "hyper-everything" (weight, cholesterol, blood pressure, diabetes, uric acid...), employed by multinationals of pharmaceuticals to test the latest-fashion molecules, presented, in postoperatory of a left inguinal hernia under general anesthesia, a right lumbar pain that was spreading in the groin. It appeared suddenly and recently and wasn't soothed by injectable paracetamol and anti-inflammatory drugs. Examining the patient, we found a plethoric abdomen, diffusely sensitive during the palpation, a painful right renal percussion, and a clean surgical bandage. The clinical evoked an ureteric colic.

Waiting for the radiological examinations, I carried out a consistent echographic examination, happy to have the opportunity to look for a dilated kidney. I was disappointed to find no kidney anomaly, but I identified an enlarged abdominal AORTA, which, in the context, meant a nonruptured aneurysm. Very discreetly, I stopped pushing the echographic probe like a frenzied on the patient's belly, as I feared I might finish the labor nature had started. The vascular surgeon was glad to have a new client!

"Knowing a patient's aorta is knowing the patient." Thus, don't deprive yourself from looking at it automatically. In transverse section from the epigastric fossa to the umbilicus, it forms a hypoechogenic circle, located in front of the lumbar spine represented by a hyperechogenic semi-circular line that creates a posterior shadow cone. On its right, the vena cava was easy to flatten, increasing the pressure of the probe. The color Doppler confirms the vascular nature.

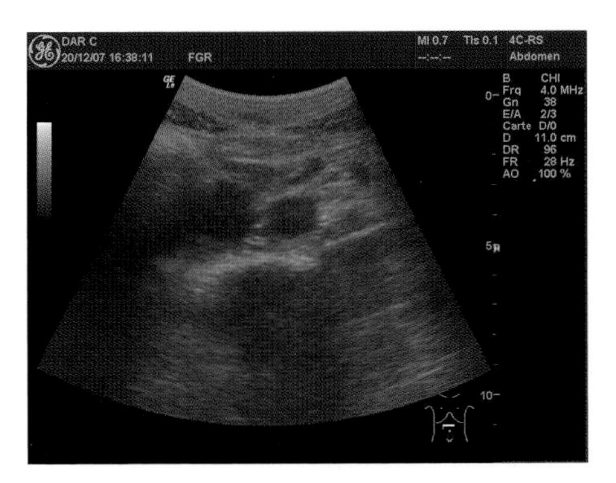

Transverse supra-umbilical section: normal inferior vena cava and abdominal aorta

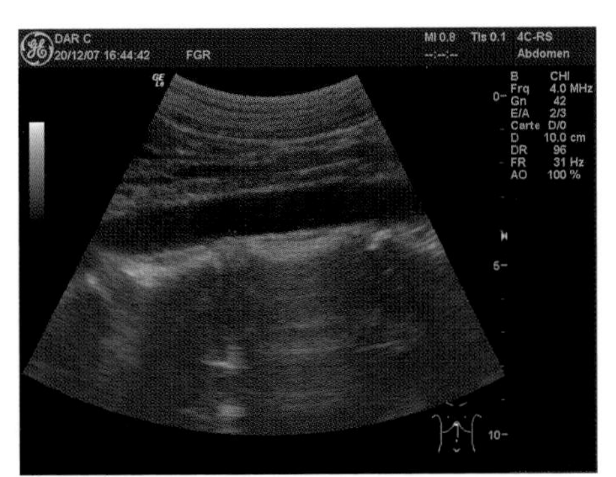

Longitudinal supra-umbilical section: normal abdominal aorta

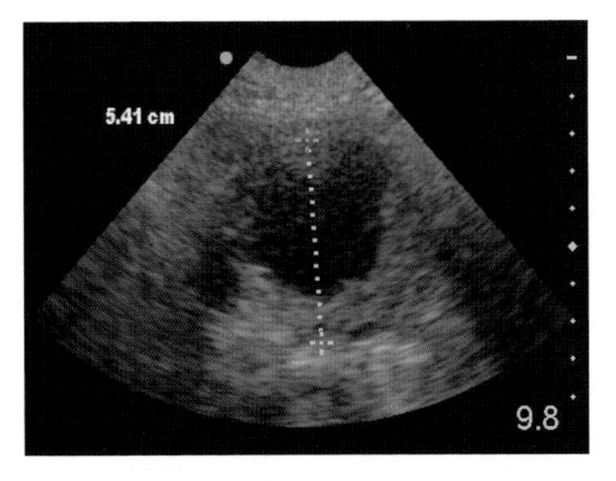

Transverse supra-umbilical section: aneurysm of abdominal aorta

We talk about aneurysm from 30 millimeters of diameter. The rotation of the probe by 90° permits to search a loss of parallelism in the walls.

To measure the aorta diameter, we just have to compare roughly the aorta diameter with the scale on the right of the screen. We can also use the "measure" menu of the echograph and place marks that appear with the trackball to measure exactly the diameter. Sometimes, the intestinal gases block the visualization of the aorta. You will have to apply a progressive and firm pressure upon the probe, which will expel the air from the intestines and permit you to see the aorta.

■ Why are you coughing?

Against his will and as he wanted to retire hurriedly, a 65-year-old man had tried to stop the latest fashionable "TRUCK" equipped with snow tires that dig trenches and fortunately not graves for our patient. As you probably suspect it, he didn't succeed. We found him intubated and ventilated in intensive care after he had been operated for a left femur fracture and sedated because of a serious cranial trauma. The third day, the nurse was worrying about the fall in prices of saturation. Closing market rate only quoted 90%. I had no stock in the Stock Exchange, so I didn't feel concerned, but I couldn't disregard it. The patient was adapted to the breathing apparatus. The pulmonary examination was normal, with maybe a little perturbation murmur at the right base, the blood pressure was still at 140/70 with a heart rate of 110 per minute, and the diuresis was 80 milliliters during the last hour; the FIO2, first at 50%, was increased to 70% in order to get the saturation back to normal. A measure of blood gas level and a thoracic x-ray were required. The thorax had not changed in comparison to the morning, and the blood gas analysis showed a 7.45 pH, an 80 mmHg PO2, and a 35 mmHg PCO2. In the morning, the PaO2 was 110 with an FIO2 of 50%.

Considering a pulmonary embolism, I watched the patient's legs without finding any obvious fact that could evoke phlebitis. I didn't know what to think and the radiologist explained to me that the scanner was a syndicated machine that only worked during daytime, so I used the echograph. I put the high-frequency linear probe on the right inguinal angle as if to search for the crural nerve, found the femoral vein, and couldn't flatten it. Watching better, I saw within the lumen a slightly hyperechogenic material. Concluding it was a right femoral phlebitis, I completed the examination exploring the popliteal fossa of the right inferior limb and the whole left inferior limb.

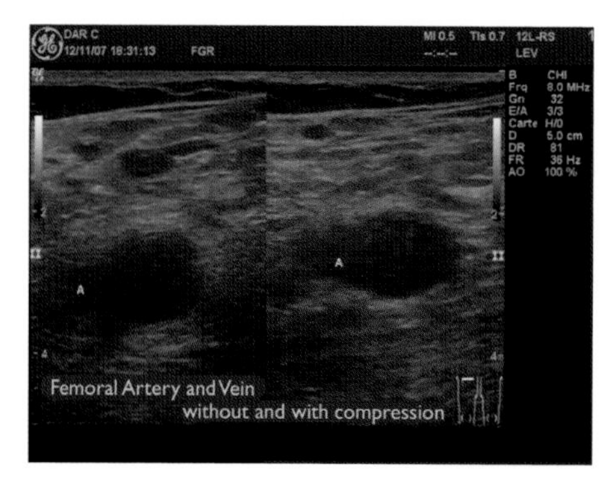

Incompressible right femoral vein

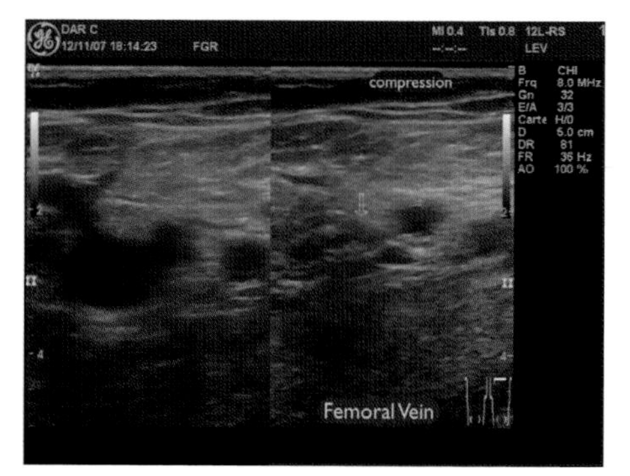

Compressible left femoral vein

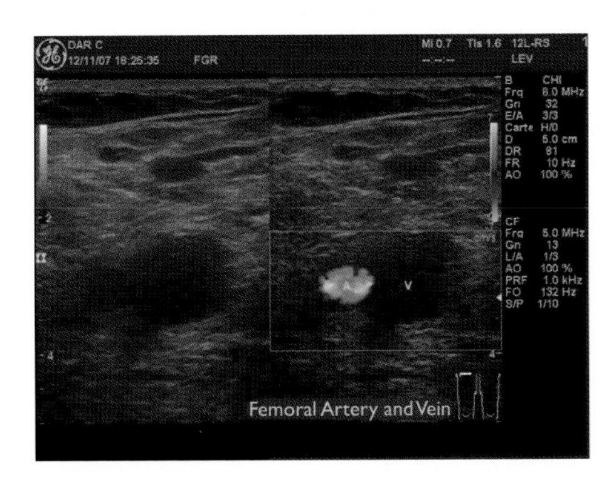

No flow in the right femoral vein (color Doppler)

With the agreement of the neurosurgeon, the orthopedic specialist, and the patient's family (I hope I forgot no one), we placed the patient under heparin. The day after, during working hours, the diagnosis of pulmonary embolism was confirmed.

Diagnosing a supra-popliteal phlebitis is very easy and can be learned very quickly. You just have to visualize femoral and popliteal veins and see whether they are compressible. Indeed, if the vein is compressible, the vein contains no thrombus, and thus there is no phlebitis. If the vein is not compressible, then follow it upwards and then downwards to look for the limits of the thrombus and check, in case of doubt, that you are really visualizing a vein finding a place where it can be flattened. For example, in the inguinal angle, you find a ganglion thinking it is the vein; it is not compressible but, when you slip the probe downwards, the image disappears.

On the contrary, the diagnosis of sub-popliteal phlebitis needs a great expertness that you will acquire with time and the help of your colleagues, specialists in vascular echography. But what is important for us is the phlebitis that can embolize, thus the supra-popliteal one.

Keep in mind that, if you suspect a pulmonary embolism, finding no supra-popliteal phlebitis never eliminates the diagnosis. Oh yes! Nothing is that simple.

Did you think about jugulars and subclavians?

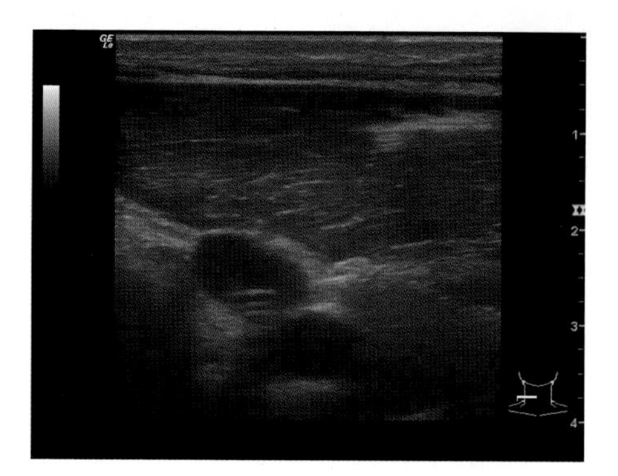

Central catheter in internal jugular, normal vein

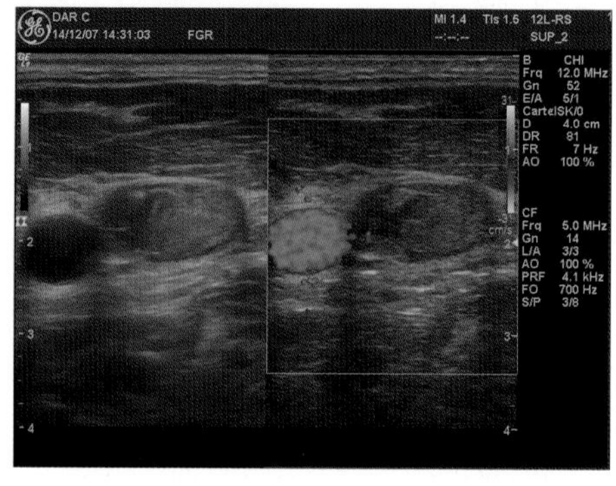

The same patient but on the other side, where a jugular catheter had previously been placed and then removed because of an unexplained hyperthermia. Internal jugular phlebitis with total thrombosis: incompressible vein, presence of visible material, and no flow

Where is it?

A 55-year-old female patient with an acute pancreatitis was brought to us from the internal medicine department to insert a central venous catheter. At first appearance, I was surprised because, usually, our colleagues from internal medicine do it themselves. But I quickly understood the trap. The conscious patient, slightly shaking, had a zest for life. I didn't need to ask her weight to estimate her BMI, which was doing well. When she understood I was the headman, she put her hands up in the air and shouted, "Oh no! Not the corrida again!". I lifted the sheet, and seeing her neck and right subclavian fossa, I understood that the banderillas had not found their way. As I was tempted to renounce giving as a pretext a last-minute emergency, the nurse immediately understood and brought me the sound machine.

I reassured the patient, telling her I was just observing her veins using a high-frequency probe. I turned the screen so she could also watch the screen. I inspected her right subclavian fossa and was surprised to see a threadlike subclavian vein and, whatever the patient's position was, this was the reason of our colleagues' disappointment. As for the left subclavian vein, it was well made, not to say plethoric. The same is for the jugulars. I showed this asymmetry to the patient. After a careful echographic tracking of the left subclavian, I put into place the central catheter without difficulty. And it is with a wide smile that the patient explained to anyone who wanted to hear that she was a left-wing woman, and she had no vein... on the right!

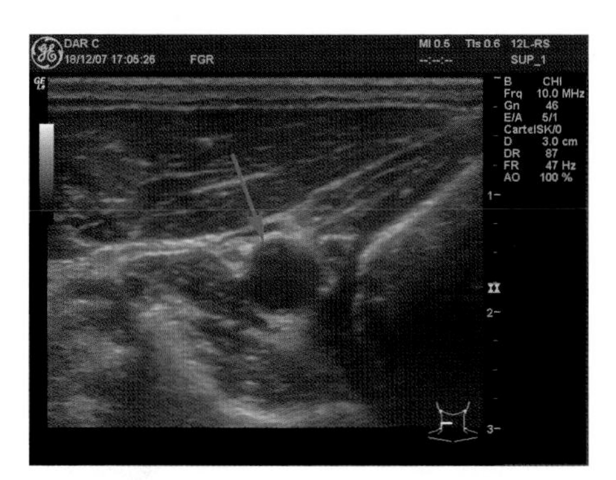

Almost inexistent right internal jugular vein, just up the right internal carotid

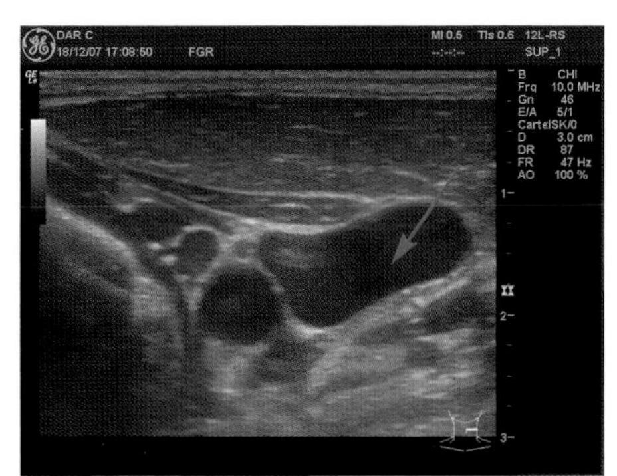

Well-visible left internal jugular vein beside the left internal carotid

"We don't need echograph to explain our success but we depend on them to explain our failures." Seeing a vein is having it. Before a puncture, marking the venous axes helps us showing the exact position of the vein, the side where the vein has the biggest diameter, and the influence of the patient's position upon its diameter and depth. These elements ensure a quick success and, anyway, avoid a puncture when the vein is missing or when it has an insignificant diameter. The echo-guidance, that is to say the puncture monitored by echography, requires a training and additional material in order to stay sterile. Try first echo-guidance for femoral or jugular vein puncture and then try the subclavian vein.

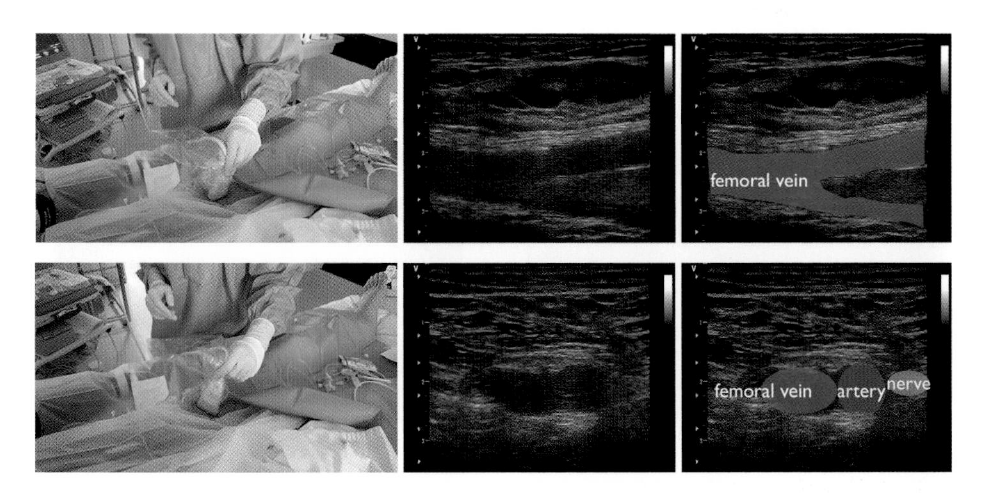

Longitudinal and transverse views of the femoral vein

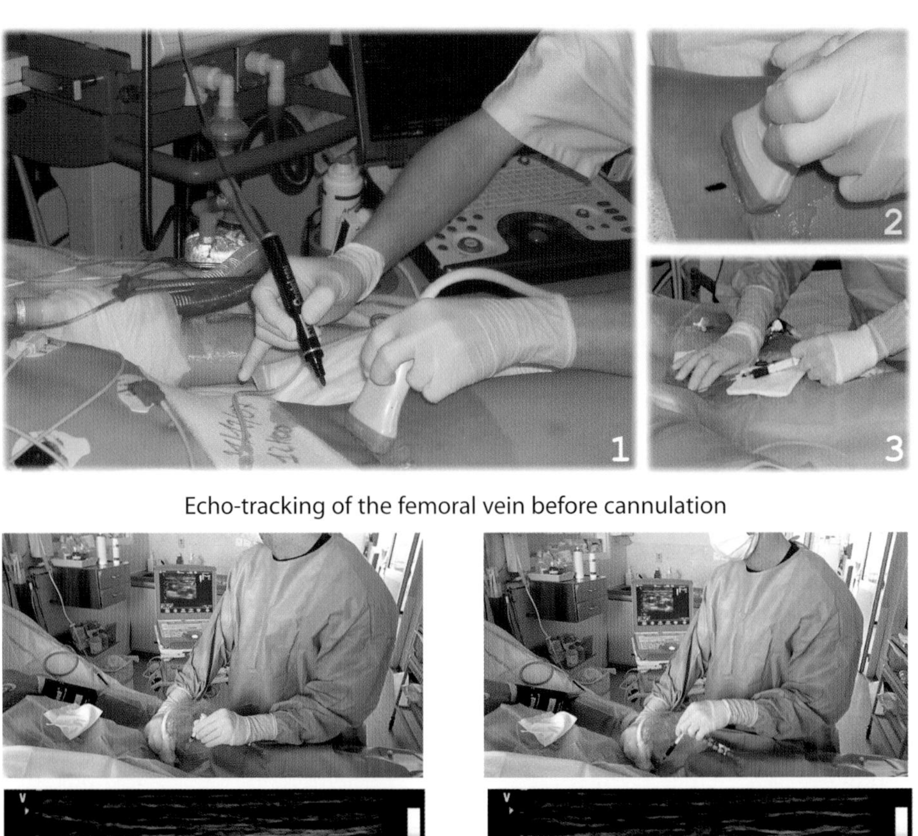

Echo-tracking of the femoral vein before cannulation

Echo-guided femoral vein cannulation (out of plane)

Just for fun, part of a letter to the editor we sent to the "Revista Española de Anestesiología y Reanimación":

Contribution of echography to Robert Aubaniac's technique to approach the subclavian vein

Although the subclavian venous catheter is the most frequently used in reanimation, only few studies describe its insertion under echography in adults.

As far as we are concerned, the main inconvenience when executing the gesture, the clavicle, is employed in order to mark more easily the subclavian vein and its puncture.

Marking the subclavian vein: After having disinfected and placed the sterile surgical drapes, a high-frequency probe is directed longitudinally according to the axis of the body. The superior edge of the probe is placed upon the internal edge of the clavicle. We scan toward the internal end of the clavicle, all the while maintaining the initial direction of the probe (1).

Thanks to this scanning, we visualize a series of longitudinal sections of subclavian surroundings, including a transverse section of the clavicle and its ultrasonic shadow. The clavicle thus represents an essential landmark. Indeed, sliding the probe, the subclavian vein emerges from the clavicle's shadow (2). It can be easily recognized, thanks to its form, its compressibility, and the presence of valves, which are sometimes visible. To make it sure, you just have to keep on scanning to make the subclavian artery appear. It has to be said that the use of color and pulsed Doppler helps to confirm but is not essential.

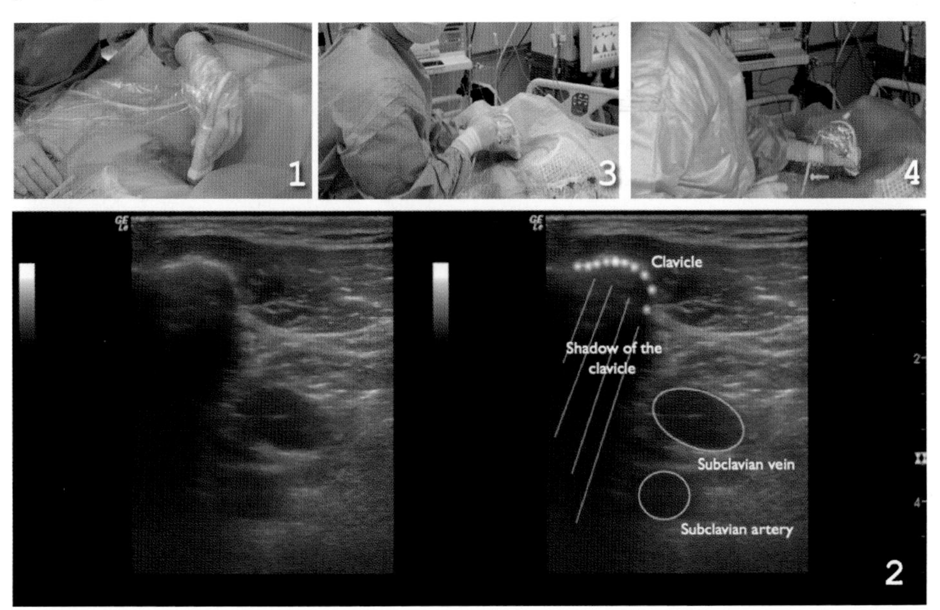

Puncture of the subclavian vein: The puncture of the vein will be executed just after its appearance from the shadow of the clavicle, where its transverse diameter is the most important. After marking the subclavian vein, the position of the probe is optimized so that this vein is placed at the center of the ultrasonographic picture. The point of puncture is out of the ultrasonic field, directly above the subclavian vein in the middle of the probe. The needle is inserted with an angle of 5° to 20° in relation to the probe's axis in an anteroposterior direction, perpendicular to the skin and parallel to the direction of the ultrasonic beam (3). The mobility of tissues permits to confirm the puncture directly above the subclavian vein and change the position of the puncture point if needed. The puncture directly above the vein permits to ensure that the needle, while moving forward, will find the vein before the thoracic structures. The relaxation of the vein, immediately followed by a blood reflux, finishes the gesture (4).

Like this, the establishment of a model to apply echography to Robert Aubaniac's technique makes not only the quick insertion of a subclavian central venous catheter in adults but also its teaching easier. Nevertheless, the use of this technique requires the previous perfect command of puncture under echography (regional anesthesia, jugular or femoral venous catheters, arterial catheterism). Finally, the absence of correct visualization of the subclavian vein can limit its use in some patients.

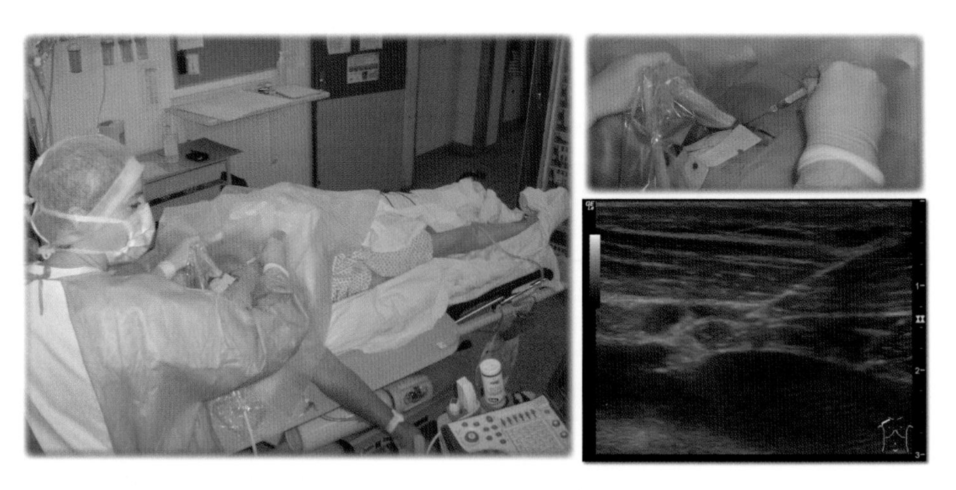

Echo-guided subclavian vein cannulation (in plane)

■ Is the center near the right or near the left?

Woken up at midnight to help a parturient to survive her pregnancy, I prepared myself for the worst, that is to say for the epidural reserved for the most arduous cases. The patient, a primiparous woman who didn't dilate in spite of wonderful contractions, seemed to need help. With the patient sitting and her back ready to receive the saving needle, I had much difficulty to find the midline. The very slender patient warned me she had gained 18 kilograms weight (39.7 lbs) along her pregnancy because of her husband, a pastry chef, who provided her with chocolate. Thanks to his flush, I immediately recognized the husband who stood apart.

I didn't want to plough her back, so I turned on the echograph that was hanging around in the labor ward. With a high-frequency probe that I held transversally, I localized the midline when I found the echographic signature of the spine, that is to say a hyperechogenic area (bone) with a shadow cone.

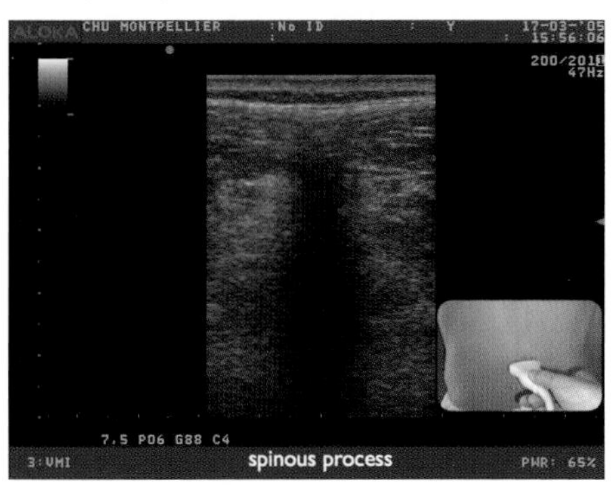

Transverse section

I marked the area turning the probe 90°. With a longitudinal section, I localized the under- and overlying spine. Asking the lady to hunch over so her back was arched, I optimized the gap between two vertebrae: interspinous process gap according to the position of the back.

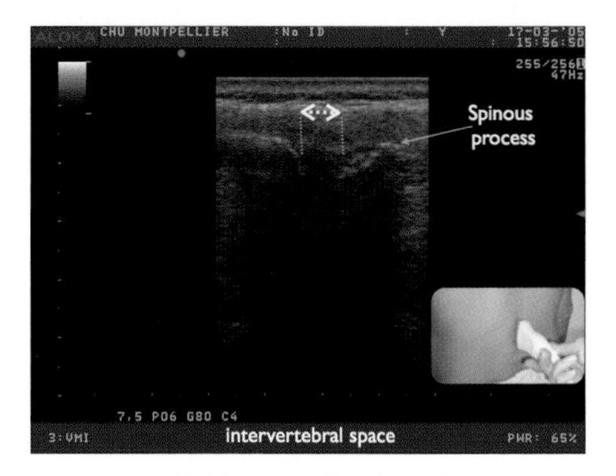

Medial longitudinal section:
back of the patient in neutral position

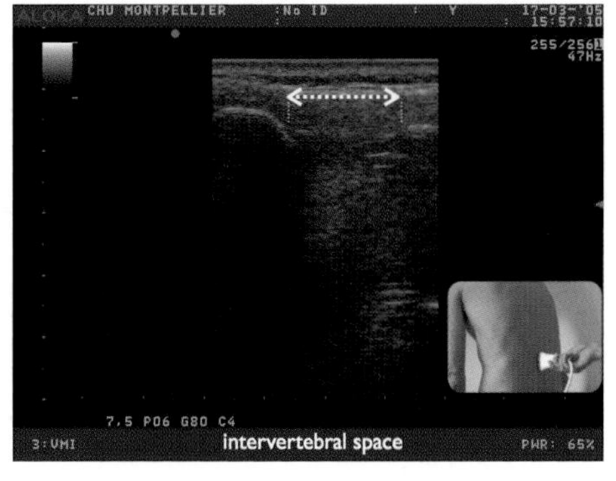

Medial longitudinal section:
patient with arched back

When this was done, I got dressed and undertook disinfection, and the gesture was brief and efficient. This didn't prevent me from waking up 2 hours later to participate in the caesarean birth.

It is obvious that we never need an echographic apparatus to carry out an epidural. But on some occasions, why should we deprive ourselves from help? Even more at 2 a.m.!

■ Tossed by the waves but is not sunk!

A 65-year-old man, loving local icefield-growing vine, has been hospitalized for 48 hours in internal medicine for an acute pancreatitis. Oh yes, another one! Going through the corridors, I was hooked by the nurse and taken to the patient who had a nocturnal dyspnea. He showed me that everything had started after the insertion of the central venous catheter in the left subclavian. The clinical examination of the patient showed a reduction of the vesicular murmur on the left with certain dullness, evoking a pleural effusion. As there was no reflux on the central catheter, the diagnosis seemed to be obvious. Armed with my low-frequency probe, I carried out the echography program, and gridding the left side, I saw the left kidney, the spleen, and, upon them, the diaphragm. Just there, unlike usually, I saw a black area without echo within which I saw, from time to time, a liver-like floating structure. Some liver in the thorax, I concluded it was hepatized lung (condensed) that was floating in some liquid. All this confirmed a left pleural effusion. The radiography required by my internist colleagues also confirmed it. The effusion was punctured with the help of an echography and gave 600 milliliters of liquid. We inserted a new central venous catheter under ultrasound guidance.

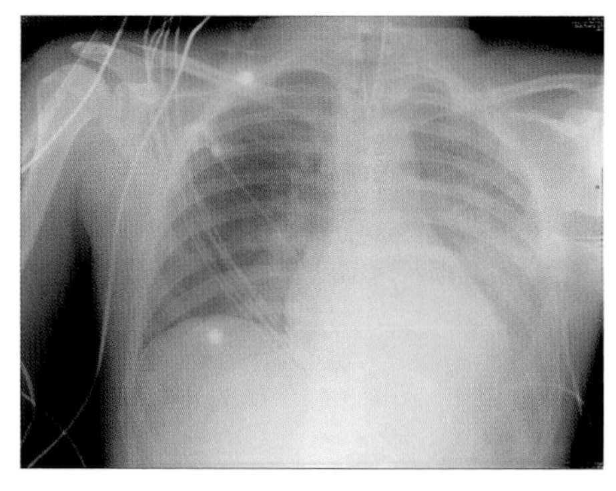

Left pleural effusion

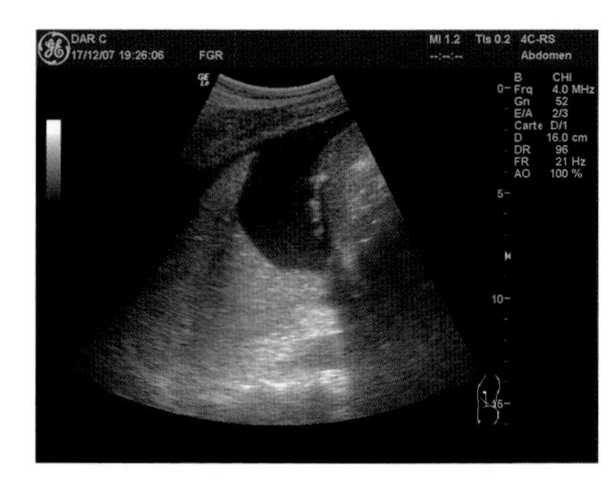

Pleural effusion with floating hepatized lung

The diagnosis of pleural effusion is easy and fast. The question is to estimate the quantity of the pleural effusion. There are many formulas to calculate the volume. But it's the clinical that gives us the solution because the real question is 'Should we puncture it?'

Effusion	+	Respiratory insufficiency	=	You should puncture
Effusion	+	Need to do bacteriologic or anatomopathological sampling	=	You should consider the puncture

The area of puncture will be determined by an echographic marking that will permit to avoid the neighboring organs.

Estimate of the effusion volume

By the way, a rough quantity estimate was suggested, thanks to a transverse section of the thorax basis with a lying patient. Once the pleural effusion is found laterally with a longitudinal section, we have to turn the probe 90° and measure on the transverse section the maximal thickness of the effusion that separates the two layers of the pleura, in millimeters. We have to multiply it by 20 to obtain a rough estimate of the volume of the pleural effusion in milliliters.

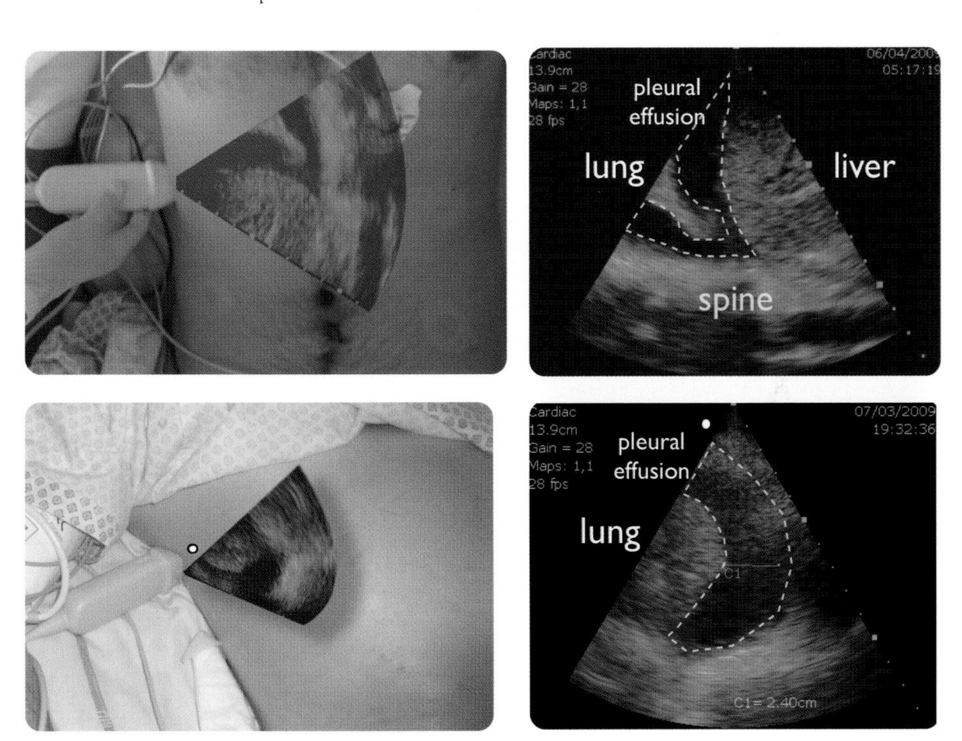

Transverse section: measurement of the pleural effusion (C1 = 24 mm). Volume of the pleural effusion in milliliters = C1 in millimeters x 20 = 24 mm x 20 = 480 ml

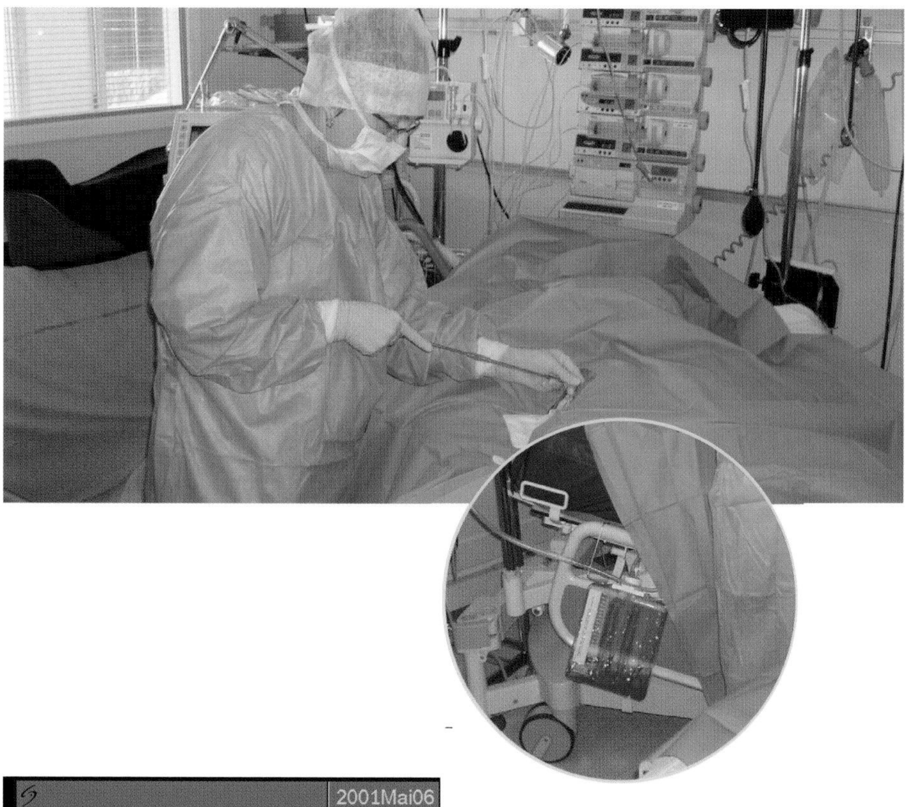

Left pleural effusion: road accident, acute respiratory insufficiency, and arterial hypertension

■ The Gordian knot?

I didn't understand why this kind 50-year-old lady, specialist in integral calculus at the French National Education, didn't manage to recover from a weight subtraction, that is to say from the exeresis of a uterine fibroma executed 4 days ago by my gynecologist colleague. She complained of indefinite abdominal pains and nausea when changing her position, all this on behalf of the resume of gases that were by the way never ending. I practiced a careful clinical examination and noticed a sensitivity of the right lumbar fossa. As the patient was not against my learning in echography, I executed a quick program of echography as a systematic habit. I was surprised to find a black area without echo and looking like a dilated renal pelvis at the level of the right kidney medulla, usually identified as echogenic (white). All this made me think of a dilatation of excretory cavities. As for the left kidney, it was normal. In this context, I called my colleague and, without any comment, showed him the knot of the problem. After an abdominal scanner, the patient was programmed for the operating room and the ureter was cleared up without a hitch.

The kidney has a very easy-to-remind echographic appearance: black periphery and white center: a real target. Thus, everything that changes this aspect must make you search for an anomaly according to the context. So don't hesitate to work on the subject; it is very profitable.

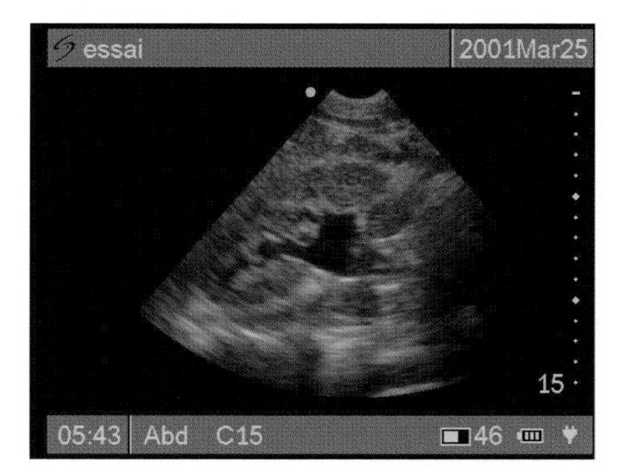

Dilatation of renal cavities

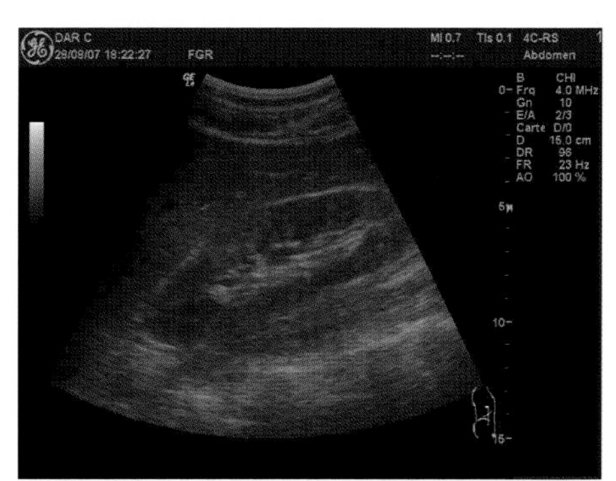

Normal kidney

■ May a woman hide another?

It was nice. Yes, it was nice outside. The thermometer indicated -20°C (-4°F). Face to this summer wave, I feared the worst. A young 25-year-old woman had fallen while she was ice-skating with her boyfriend. When we took charge of her, she had a cranial trauma with an occipital wound. The patient opened her eyes when we asked her and spoke with incomprehensible words; she had reactivity in flexion adapted to the neurostimulation. Her Glasgow score was 10. Carefully turbaned after we had placed a cervical collar, the patient was admitted to the emergency department. The clinical examination showed nothing more. According to her boyfriend, the patient had no noticeable antecedent and took no treatment. Waiting for a cerebral and cervical scanner, we carried out a training echographic examination. We stopped a while on the third step, the one that looks for liquid in the Douglas pouch. Our eyes were attracted by the presence of a third-type element within the uterus: the Miss was a Mrs. We took the necessary measures of x-ray protection. The β-HCG confirmed our vision.

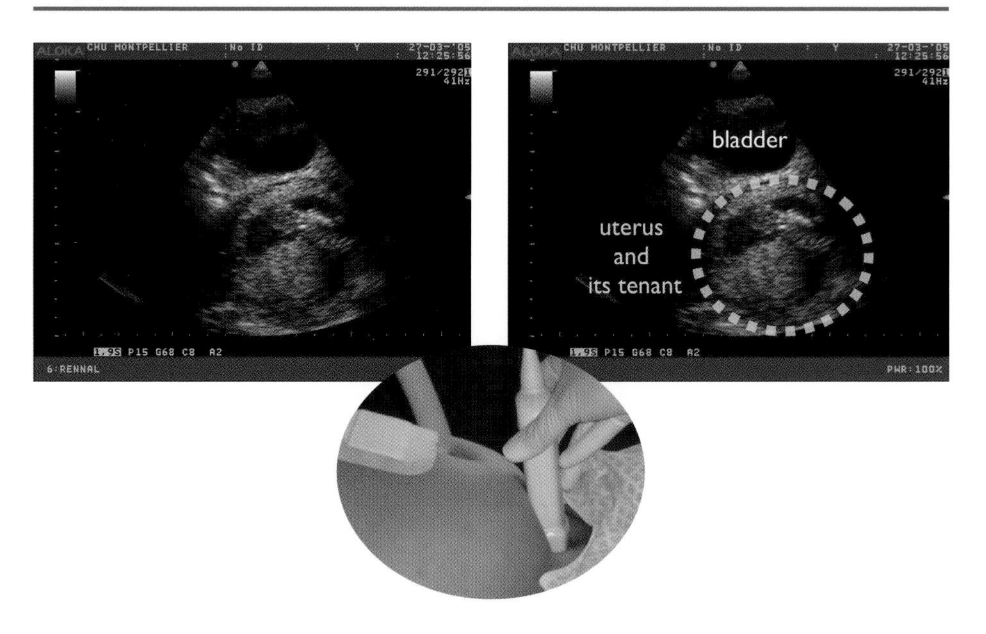

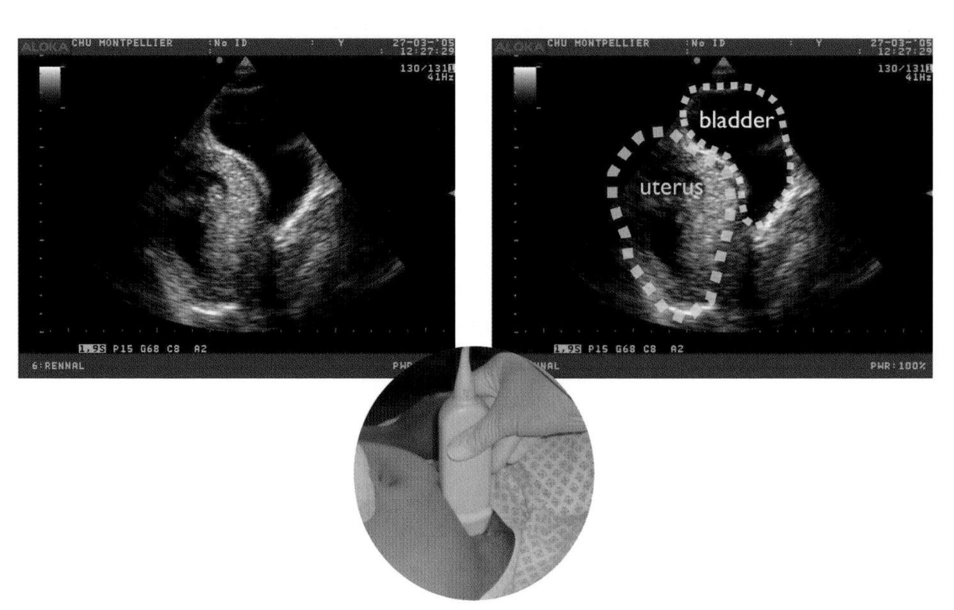

Obvious pregnancy. Everybody knows, except us!

The echography doesn't permit to eliminate the possibility of an intra-uterine pregnancy. We have to wait for the 6th or 7th week of amenorrhea to bring to light an intra-uterine egg by abdominal way. On the contrary, the echography permits to warn rapidly if something is visible in the uterus. We will use this information according to the context and the dosage of β-HCG.

■ It's not a good calculus

"Doctor, remove this damned gallbladder. It makes my life unbearable." The cry was so loud that it woke me up. I tried to fall back asleep, but was shaken again out of my dreams by this supplication that seemed to come out from beyond the grave. Infuriated, I got out of the rest room, followed the way of the sound wave, and eventually came across my emergency colleague grappling with a "stout" kind lady as red as a beetroot by dint of belting out claiming for the sacrificial gift of her gallbladder on the altar of surgery. She explained that her belly hurt and it was her gallbladder. She had read it in the paper at her hairdresser's.

The clinical examination showed a distended stomach, painful in a diffuse way. We noticed hydroaeric noises. The patient was apyretic. At her side, her husband, very civil, waited patiently for my colleague's verdict, hoping, you never know, a certain relief.

Skeptical, my colleague asked me to assist him and took the echograph while waiting for our radiologist colleague. After a consistent examination of clarification that showed no obvious anomaly, we concentrated on the right hypochondrium. With the longitudinal section of Morison, we located the inferior edge of the liver; my colleague easily found an anechogenic pouch under the liver with a pear shape and a posterior reinforcement. The color Doppler didn't show any blood flow. It was obviously the gallbladder. By movements of translation, the whole gallbladder was explored and no calculus was found. (A calculus can be easily located because it's a hyperechogenic area with a posterior shadow cone). Moreover, the pressure of the probe on the gallbladder wasn't particularly painful. The absence of gallstone and the absence of any echographic sign of Murphy confirmed our clinical feeling: the patient had to keep her gallbladder! The radiologist also confirmed our point of view and the patient was clearly improved, thanks to a prescription of Buscopan. Oh yes! Her spasmodic colitis had once again won the game.

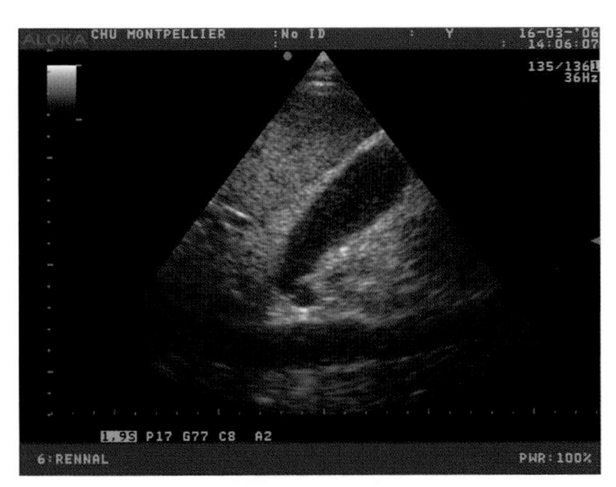

Longitudinal section on the right midclavicular line under the costal edge: gallbladder with, in the background, the inferior vena cava

The diagnosis of cholecystitis is a hard one in echography for beginners, particularly in reanimation. The pain when you run the echographic transducer upon the gallbladder, or echographic sign of Murphy, is a meaningful sign, but other criteria of ultrasound diagnosis such as "wall thickened of more than 4 millimeters, heterogeneous wall, peri-vesicular effusion, big gallbladder, presence of a calculus" are not very specific elements and we can find them on any patient of reanimation without them having an acute cholecystitis.

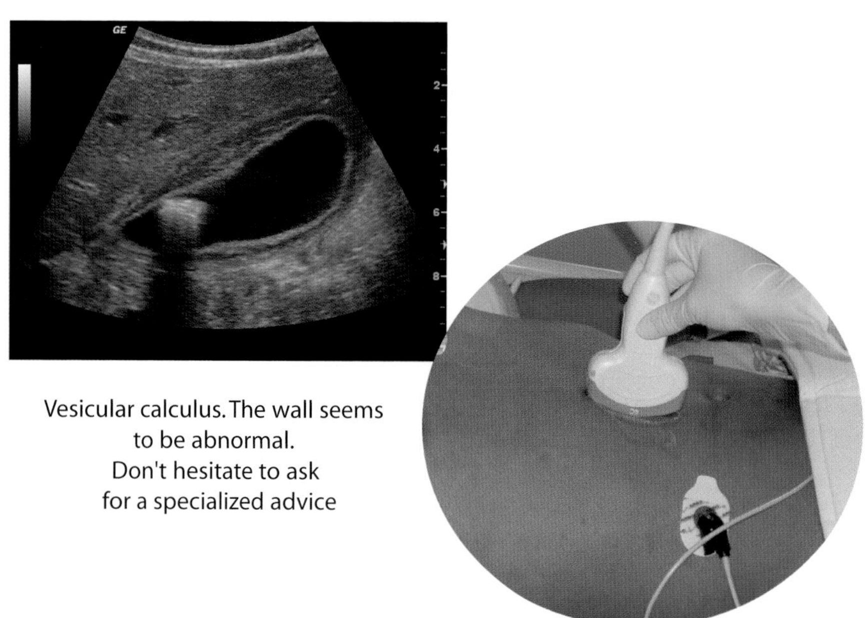

Vesicular calculus. The wall seems to be abnormal.
Don't hesitate to ask for a specialized advice

On the contrary, when there is no pain when you run the probe and when there is no visualized calculus, the negative predictive value is 98%. Thus the echography, even for a beginner, permits, after a careful examination, to confirm there is a little probability of having an acute cholecystitis and then to start looking for another pathology.

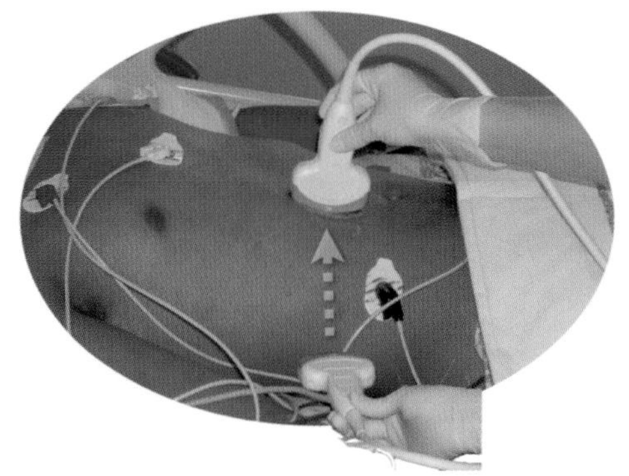

Searching the gallbladder from the section of Morison's pouch by lateral way

Conclusion

The first winter I spent on the ice field permitted me to become acquainted with the world of echography: incredible tool that allows you to see, beyond the skin, the internal difference. Conscious of my ignorance I consulted books, studied scanners, and attended presentations of my radiologist colleague, to eventually realize that the best echographic examination was worth nothing without a good clinical examination.

The essentials to learn

■ Echography and emergency room

The quick evolution of technology permitted to develop and produce compact echographs, suited to the necessities of emergency medicine and the hospital budgets. Now that the machines are available, we have to learn how to use them well.

An **academic training, given by experts in medical imaging**, cannot be avoided to become an ultrasonographer and master every aspect of reference echography. In the continuation of our topic, we will get onto the learning methods and the use of an echograph in an emergency room by nonradiologist doctors. This echography of clarification, as it is called, represents a continuation of the clinical examination and rapidly answers accurate questions that could direct the patient to the right care unit.

On December 4, 1997, a consensus conference [1] took place in Baltimore, USA, in order to establish recommendations about the use of ultrasound by surgeons when taking care of patients who are victims of a traumatism. The FAST, Focused Assessment with Sonography for Trauma, was born. This examination aims at searching and highlighting the presence of an intra-abdominal or pericardial effusion, in a quick way and without delaying the initial measures for resuscitation. It consists in the echographic exploration of the four regions (the "**4P**": 1, Pericardial; 2, Perihepatic; 3, Perisplenic; 4, Pelvis) where we look for a liquid effusion visualized with a black area without echo. With time and according to the authors, we also added the detection of other elements such as thoracic liquid or gaseous effusions and aneurysms of the abdominal aorta.

The recommendations about the minimum formation were 8 hours of teaching, split into 4 hours of theory and 4 hours of practical works, completing the whole with the execution of at least 200 overseen examinations before being considered as autonomous. Since then, several authors diminished the number of necessary examinations. Tso *et al.* [2] use an hour of theory combined with an hour of practice with a sensitivity of 91% and a specificity of 96% out of 163 patients studied in a prospective way. Rocycki *et al.* [3] developed a course of 32 hours of instruction with a sensitivity of 83% and a specificity of 99% out of a total of 1540 patients. The study of the learning curve made by Ma *et al.* [4] highlighted the need of doing at least 50 overseen examinations. Smith *et al.* [5] established that 25 examinations were enough, and Shackford *et al.* [6] concluded that 10 examinations were enough to execute the FAST correctly. Even better, McCarter *et al.* [7] had no learning curve.

These different studies seem to show the efficiency of a limited initial formation in echography for this precise context, all the more so as the results obtained by surgeons or radiologists were quite similar when executing the FAST [8, 9], or became so with experience [10, 11]. Since 1997, the use of ultrasounds in traumatology is part of the Advance Trauma Life Support (ATLS) course taught by the American College of Surgeons.

Thus, the FAST represents, obviously and with proofs, the unavoidable base to teach any doctor who wants to use an echograph in emergency department. It appears that a theoretical and practical teaching of 8 hours in total is the minimum acknowledged in order to obtain one's echographic driving license. Nevertheless, we are surprised to see that the study of literature doesn't permit to define exactly the contents of these 8 hours. Han *et al.* [12], as well as Sisley *et al.* [13], draw the outlines of these contents but their studies don't permit to have a sufficiently accurate idea to apply it simply.

Thus it is difficult for us to talk about learning methods of echography in emergency department from the data collected in the literature. We have to admit that what will follow is nothing else than a try, comforted by on-the-job experience, to throw the bases of a thinking about the structure of a learning method for the FAST. To date, there is no truth about this topic.

An echographic examination in an emergency situation made by an emergency doctor includes several special features that we have to take into consideration:

Time: When the vital process is threatened, a special dimension appears: time, and thus every minute matters. Thus, the echographic examination must be carried out within a maximum period, which we will arbitrarily set on 3 minutes (ideal time of resistance of cerebral cells in hypoxia).

Stress: It is provoked by the situation of emergency, lack of time, fear of not being good enough when doing the echography, other people's opinion, and so on.

Technical flexibility: The emergency doctor can, according to circumstances, be part of various operation situations due to his transversality (particularly during the night) and then be confronted with the use of various echographic machines that he will have to actuate on his own.

Confusion of roles: The emergency doctor and the radiologist have two different, complementary roles: the former takes charge of the patient and is a decision-maker; the latter has an advisory role when pronouncing an echographic diagnosis, all the while letting the emergency doctor insert it in his clinical practice. When the emergency doctor carries the echographic examination out, he is judge and party at the same time. And this can affect the acuity of his echographic examination.

Low exposure: The echographic activity of an emergency doctor is minor in comparison to the radiologist's. The method must be simple and at the same time have a strong endurance to resist to time.

We also have to consider the fact that, as an echographic examination is a manual gesture, it is the result of a motor skill. Doctor Desmurget, a neurophysiologist [14], reminds us that the exact imitation of a gesture done by the teacher can be done by the apprentice only if the pupil has a precise knowledge of the shape his body takes during the action. And yet, this knowledge only comes from training. The learning process of the gesture can only be achieved through direct confrontation with the task; showing it doesn't pass on information about the dynamic properties of movement.

Thus, the mission is to learn, in 8 hours' time, how to make four specific pictures from the echographic exploration of four areas of the abdomen and how to interpret them and consider their use in the clinical situation, within a specific time context, a given working atmosphere, with different echographs, and having to immediately assume the result of one's examination.

In the action, body and mind must form a whole. The thought becomes the gesture, and the gesture becomes action exactly when all the knowledge is drawn together. In order to be efficient, the action, submitted to the pressure of time, must have a logical chain and a sensible management based upon an operative pattern. This pattern must already exist in thought and not be invented or reinvented during each situation. This represents the whole interest of acquired experience: this is where the learning process must lie, with as goal the passing of knowledge, but above all, of a know-how [15].

Thus, during these 8 hours of teaching, we have to train tirelessly the learner on the practical fulfillment of a series of elementary processes that constitute an operative program resulting from the synthesis of indispensable knowledge and the establishment of a pattern from the practice of experts. This forms a Fast Program of Echography.

The program sets a real path punctuated with steps with a precise goal: making a characteristic photograph of the explored area. The path begins on the right side, and then the left side and the hypogastrium, the thorax, and the upper abdomen to finish in the inguinal angle.

Thus, learning the path can be done in five units of study (described in the self-training procedure), integrating into the FAST the observation of pleurae, aorta and the vena cava. Each step has a specific goal. The study of the right side permits to find Morison's pouch [16] (inter-hepatorenal space) and take a photo looking for a liquid effusion between the liver and the kidney. At the same time, the perihepatic

Learning each step starts with the presentation of the essential knowledge in 20 minutes, which is then put into practice in an hour. The theoretical course is based upon the presentation of the normal picture to be found, the pathological picture and a few variations, the video of a normal examination, and the video of a pathological examination. The bases of ultrasounds are progressively taught and repeated all along the 8 hours.

The practical works are done by three-student groups around an echograph. An instructor overlooks two groups of students.

Each pupil successively plays the patient (he feels and sees the result of the position of the probe and the movement on his body, which is a visual and kinesthetic programming), the doctor (he sees and feels the result of the position of the probe, feeling sadness or satisfaction according to the result, which is a visual and kinesthetic programming), and the witness (separated from the situation, he can talk freely about what he's seeing, which is an auditory and visual programming). This way, the pupil memorizes the process looking, feeling, and talking about what he's doing. He thinks, does, and teaches, and thus the learning process is total [17, 18].

Each step includes a subprogram that permits, in 100% of cases, when it is possible, to obtain the set goal without knowledge in anatomy, without thinking, just following the program. This is called "gridding"; it is an exploration of the area made according to a consistent longitudinal scanning searching for a defined target, easy to recognize. **Executing this consistent process in less than 5 minutes, the beginner finds, in any case, Morison's pouch. The same is for the other steps.**

The obvious easiness with which the pupil, without any previous knowledge of echography, can find Morison's pouch (thing he had never dreamed of when registering for this course) positively reinforces him and makes the continuation of learning much simpler.

The printed photo is then stuck onto a learning booklet so that the learner makes his own study book.

When he carries out the next step, we ask the student to start with the previous steps before doing the new one; it obliges him to start again and again from the beginning. At the end of the 8 hours, each pupil will have repeated the process at least 15 times.

A standardized examination report completes the process. The doctor is trained to answer to specific questions; it defines the object of the examination, thanks to YES, NO, or I DON'T KNOW [1].

The pupil is assessed with an initial and final theoretical examination [13] and a final practical examination made on a healthy subject. The goal is to make the five basic pictures in less than 4 minutes.

The pupil is assessed with an initial and final theoretical examination [13] and a final practical examination made on a healthy subject. The goal is to make the five basic pictures in less than 4 minutes.

This course, which began at the initiative of the magazine "Urgence Pratique" [19], has the advantage of being easy to put into place; it can put up with the training of a large number of doctors, it takes account of the constraints of practicing echography in emergency medicine, and it permits to answer the following questions in less than 4 minutes:

Is there a liquid or gas effusion in the abdomen?
Is there a liquid or gas effusion in the pleura?
Is there a pericardial effusion?
Does the heart beat? Has he got a good contraction?
Is there a visible vesicular lithiasis?
Is there an aneurysm of the abdominal aorta?
Is there an obvious pregnancy?
Is there urinary tract dilatation?
Is there a dilatation of the urinary bladder?
What is the diameter of the vena cava?
Where are the jugulars, subclavian, and femoral vessels?
(And secondarily besides the given time:
Is there a femoropopliteal phlebitis?)

An advantage of its conception is that the course is only based upon five pictures and one gesture, "gridding", which form a method of self-instruction. As he is programmed to find a normal anatomy, the doctor can, if he has an echograph at his disposal, train at leisure and thereby maintain his know-how over time.

At the end of the training, out of more than 1500 trained doctors, 100% of doctors manage to carry out the entire process in less than 4 minutes on a healthy subject.

A thesis, defended in 2005 at the Faculté de Médecine of Montpellier in France to obtain the rank of doctor in medicine, prospectively assesses for a period of 6 months the use of echography in abdominal traumatisms in the emergency department of the Hôpital Saint-Paul on Reunion Island [20]. All the doctors of the unit had been trained with the fast program of echography and used a HP Sonos 2000. Out of 39 patients with a closed abdominal traumatism, the sensitivity of the examination was 71%, the specificity reached 100%, the positive predictive value was 100%, and the negative predictive value was 93%. These results confirm those from literature and can form the beginning of a proof of the efficiency of the training made only on a healthy subject.

The congresses and trips permit to realize that the different training courses for echography in emergency department are not very different basically. The main difference lies within the learning models. Our Anglo-Saxon colleagues gladly suggest

Altogether, technology permits us to benefit from the echographic tools on the patient's bed and a quick training permits us to use them well. This training course is based upon an ancestral methodology that regulates the learning of a manual gesture: practice makes perfect!

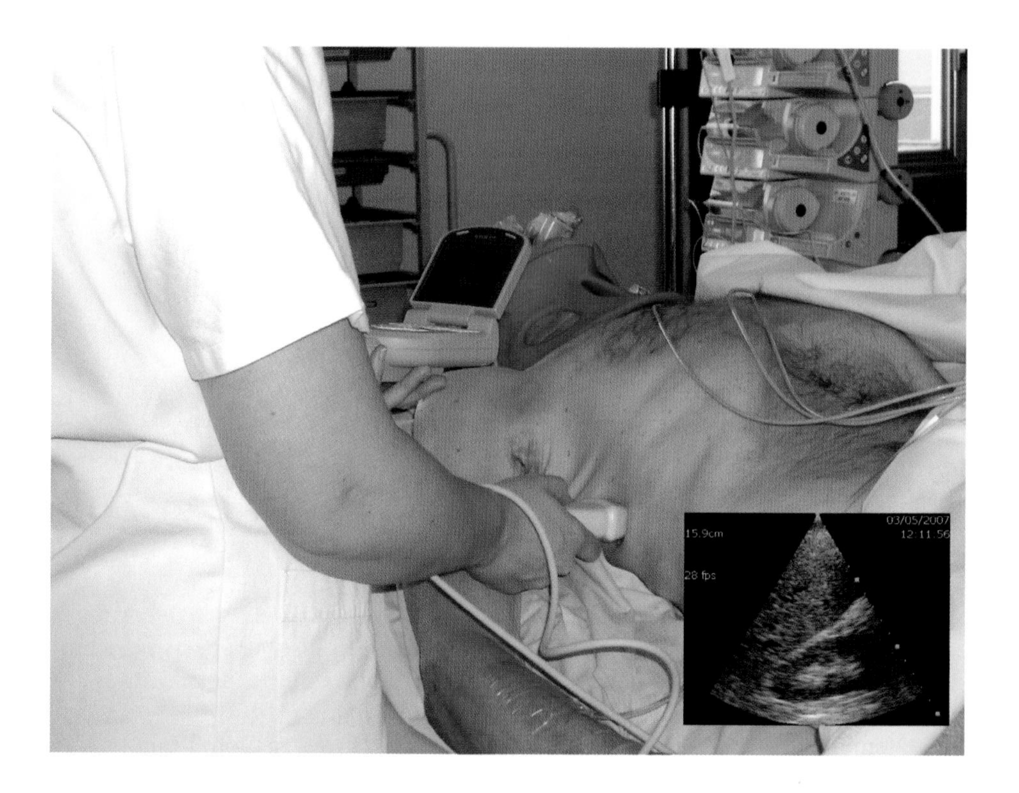

References

1 - Scalea TM, Rodriguez A, Chiu WC, Brenneman FD, Fallon WF, Kato K, McKenney MG, Nerlich ML, Ochsner MG, Yoshii H. Focused assessment with sonography for trauma (FAST): results from an international consensus conference. J Trauma. 1999; 46: 466-72

2 - Tso P, Rodriguez A, Cooper C *et al.* Sonography in blunt abdominal trauma: a preliminary progress report. J Trauma. 1992; 33: 39-44

3 - Rozycki GS, Ochsner MG, Jaffin JH, Champion HR. Prospective evaluations of surgeons' use of ultrasound in the evaluation of trauma patients. J Trauma. 1993; 34: 516-27

4 - Ma OJ, Mateer JR, Ogata M, Kefer MP, Wittmann D, Aprahamian C. Prospective analysis of rapid trauma ultrasound examination performed by emergency physicians. J Trauma. 1995; 38: 879-85

5 - Smith RS, Kern SJ, Fry WR, Helmer ST. Institutional learning curve of surgeon-performed trauma ultrasound. Arch Surg. 1998; 133: 530-3

4 - Ma OJ, Mateer JR, Ogata M, Kefer MP, Wittmann D, Aprahamian C. Prospective analysis of rapid trauma ultrasound examination performed by emergency physicians. J Trauma. 1995; 38: 879-85
5 - Smith RS, Kern SJ, Fry WR, Helmer ST. Institutional learning curve of surgeon-performed trauma ultrasound. Arch Surg. 1998; 133: 530-3
6 - Shackford SR, Rogers FB, Osler TM, Trabulsy ME, Claus DW, Vane DW. Focused abdominal sonogram for trauma: the learning curve of nonradiologist clinicians in detecting hemoperitoneum. J Trauma. 1999; 46: 553-62
7 - McCarter FD, Luchette FA, Molloy M, Hurst JM, Davis K, Johannigman JA, Frame SB, Fischer JE. Institutional and individual learning curves for focused abdominal ultrasound for trauma. Ann Surg. 2000; 231: 689-700
8 - McKenney MG, McKenney KL, Compton RP *et al.* Can surgeons evaluate emergency ultrasound scans for blunt abdominal trauma? J Trauma. 1998; 44: 649-53
9 - Buzzas GR, Kern SJ, Smith RS, Harrison PB, Helmer SD, Reed JA. A comparison of sonographic examinations for trauma performed by surgeons and radiologists. J Trauma. 1998; 44: 604-6
10 - Förster R, Pillasch J, Zielke A, Malewski U, Rothmund M. Ultrasonography in blunt abdominal trauma: influence of the investigators' experience. J Trauma. 1992; 34: 264-9
11 - Thomas B, Falcone RE, Vasquez D *et al.* Ultrasound evaluation of blunt abdominal trauma: program implementation, initial experience, and learning curve. J Trauma. 1997; 42: 384-8
12 - Han D, Rozycki GS, Schmidt JA, Feliciano D: Ultrasound training during ATLS: an early start for surgical interns. J Trauma. 1996; 41: 208-13
13 - Sisley AC, Johnson SB, Erickson WRN, Fortune JBD: Use of an Objective Structured Clinical Examination (OSCE) for the assessment of physician performance in the ultrasound evaluation of trauma. J Trauma. 1999; 47: 627-32
14 - Desmurget M. Imitation et apprentissages moteurs: des neurones miroirs à la pédagogie du geste sportif. Solal éditeur, Marseille - 2006
15 - Pitti R. Formation des médecins de proximité. Urgences Pratique. 1998; 26: 29-32
16 - Morison R. The anatomy of the right hypochondrium relating especially to operations for gallstones. Br Med J 1894; 2: 968
17 - La Garanderie ADE. Pédagogie des moyens d'apprendre. Le Centurion, Paris 1989
18 - La Garanderie ADE. Profils pédagogiques. Le Centurion, Paris 1980
19 - Greco F. Echographie : que la main du médecin fasse ! Urgence Pratique. 2003; 56: 57-8
20 - Tournan V. L'échographie devant un traumatisme abdominal : utilisation du PREP (Programme Rapide d'Échographie du Polytraumatisé) aux urgences de Saint-Paul de La Réunion. Thèse d'exercice : Médecine : Montpellier 1: 2005
21 - Abu-Zidan FM, Siöstenn AK, Wang J, Al-Ayoubi F, Lennquist S. Establishment of a teaching animal model for sonographic diagnosis of trauma. J Trauma. 2004; 56: 99-104
22 - Knudson MM, Sisley A. Training residents using simulation technology: experience with ultrasound trauma. J Trauma. 2000

Self-training procedure

■ In order to fulfill your reading, put your hand on the probe

You have to make the five elementary pictures of the program and paste them in the book on the places reserved for that purpose. Take part in the play and you will be pleasantly surprised at the result.

STEP 1: Look for the right kidney and Morison's pouch

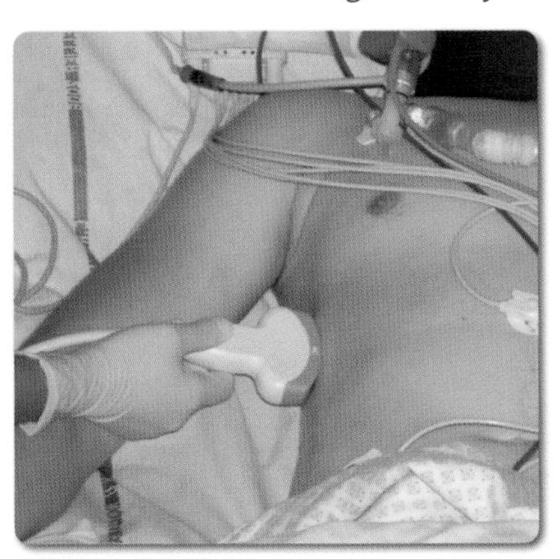

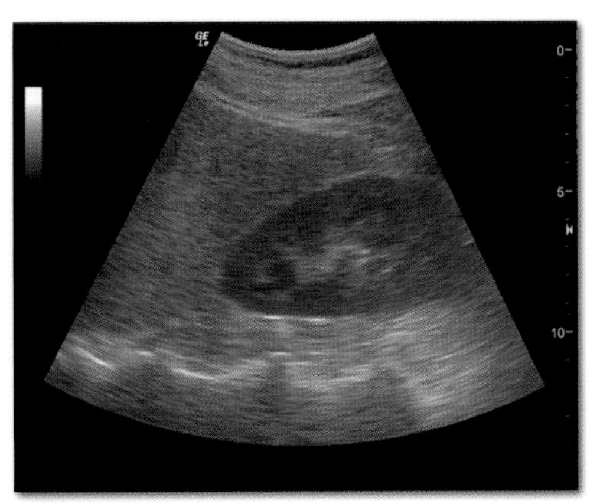

STEP I

- If you can, place yourself on the patient's right with the echograph.
- Plug the machine in, if necessary.
- Turn the machine on, pushing the on/off button.
- Select a low-frequency probe, preferably an abdominal one, and connect it to the machine.
- Check the probe cleanliness; if need be, wipe it with adequate wipes.
- Check that the probe works well by applying gel. If nothing happens on the screen, check the connection or unfreeze the image by pushing the "GEL" button.
- Check depth: minimum 12 centimeters. Not being sure, set it on the maximum.
- Make sure the image mark is on the left of the screen. If need be, touch one end of the probe with your finger and observe the symmetry on the screen.
- With the probe mark toward the patient's head, put the probe longitudinally on the anterior axillary line opposite to the nipple.

- Slide the probe along the anterior axillary line toward the patient's feet, while at the same time keeping the probe parallel to the bed.
- Watch the screen, and if you don't see the kidney along the anterior axillary line, do the same movement again on the medium axillary line, and then on the posterior one until you identify the kidney.
- Once you have located Morison's pouch, freeze the image, print it, paste it, and comment it.

Paste your picture here

STEP 2: Find the left kidney

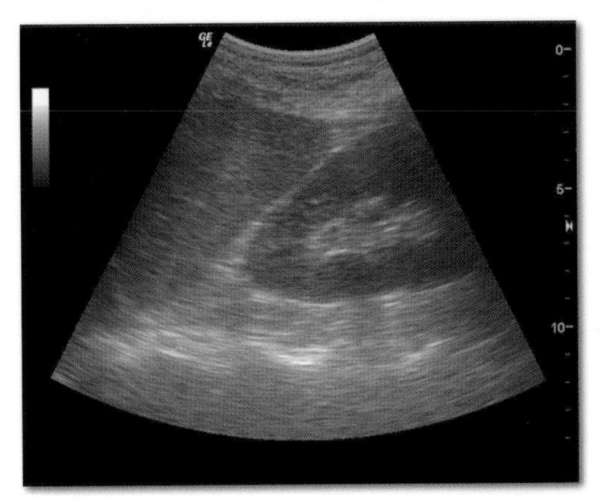

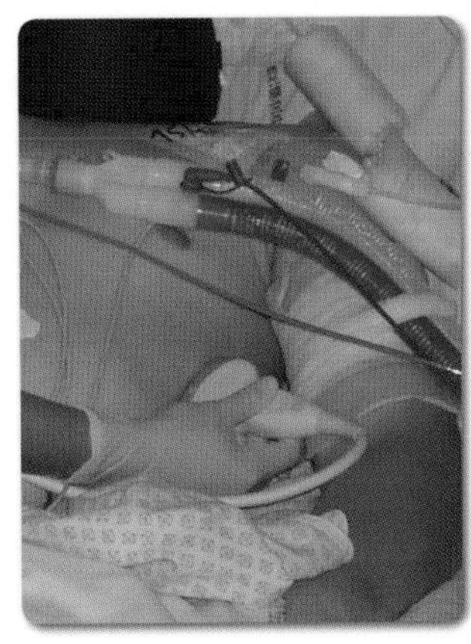

STEP 2

- Before you proceed to the second step, just for fun, do the first step again.
- Same gestures as in the step #1, but this time, put the probe on the left anterior axillary line. The left kidney is generally higher and more posterior than the right kidney. Thus, don't hesitate to grid as far as the bed's level.
- Once the left kidney is identified, mobilize the probe in order to visualize the space between the inferior edge of the spleen and the superior pole of the kidney. Freeze the image, print it, paste it, and comment it.

Paste your picture here

STEP 3: Find the bladder

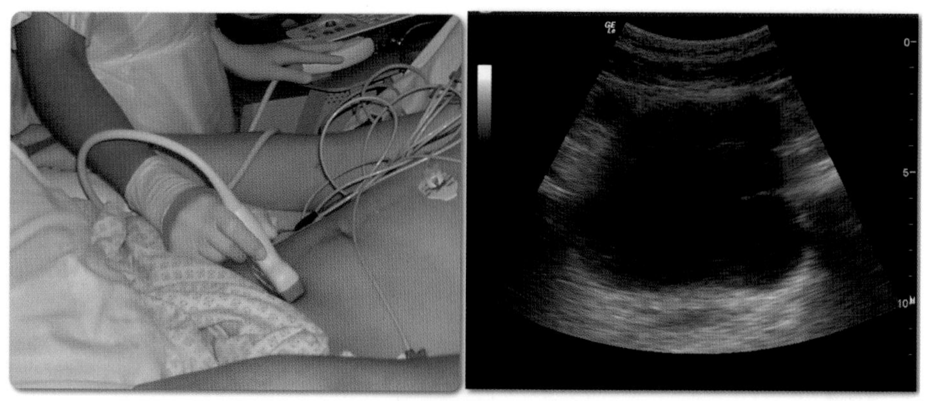

STEP 3

- Do the steps #1 and #2 before proceeding to step #3.
- With the probe's mark toward the patient's head, put the probe longitudinally on the medium subumbilical line.
- Slide the probe downwards until you bump into the pubis.
- If need be, direct the transducer toward the patient's feet in order to visualize the bladder.
- Turn the probe 90° counter-clockwise in order to direct the probe's mark toward the patient's right.
- Visualize the bladder in transverse section.
- Freeze the image, print it, paste it, and comment it.

Paste your picture here

STEP 4: Find the heart

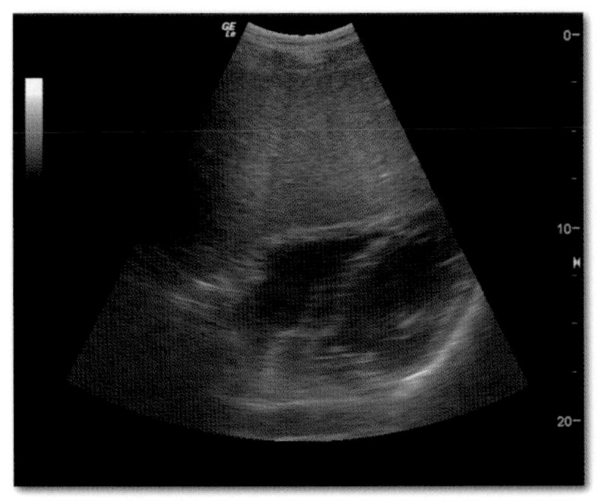

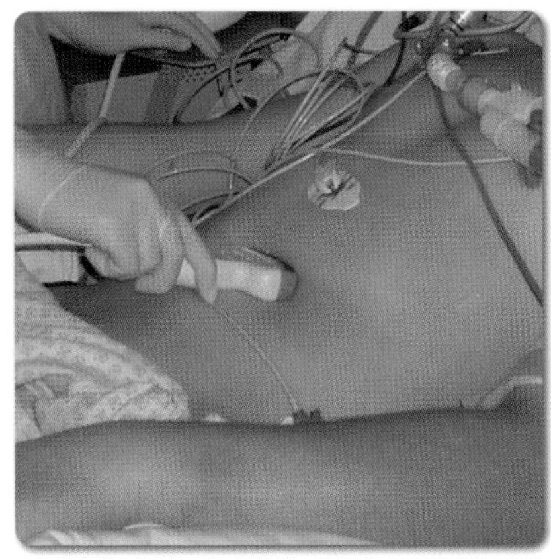

STEP 4

- Oh yes! Once again, do the first steps before starting the fourth one.
- Increase depth: set it on 20 centimeters.
- With the probe's mark toward the patient's right, put the probe transversally in the epigastric fossa and direct it toward the right shoulder of the patient.
- Apply a pressure to sink the transducer under the level of costal edge. The probe must be almost parallel to the skin.
- If you don't see something moving progressively, turn the probe keeping it flat, toward the right shoulder of the patient until you can see the heart in motion.
- Freeze the image, print it, and comment it.
- In case of failure, do the opposite gesture toward the left shoulder, leaning the transducer 20° upwards to see deeper. You can ask the patient to fold his knees in order to relax the abdominal wall.
- If, nevertheless, you don't manage to see the heart, proceed to next step. (Actually, when the heart cannot be seen from down below, it is clearly visible by executing a left parasternal longitudinal thoracic gridding.)

Paste your picture here

STEP 5: Find the aorta

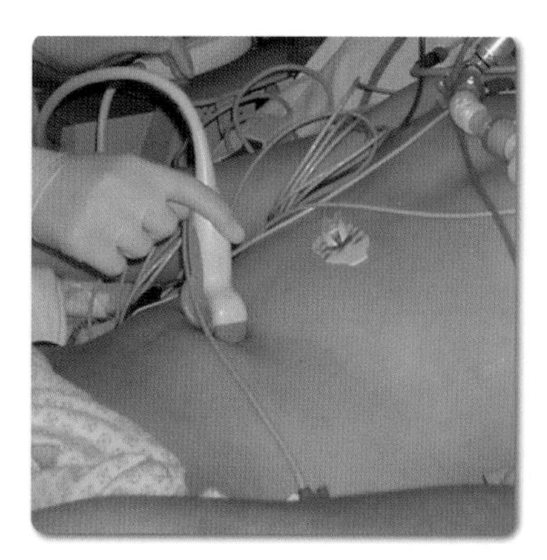

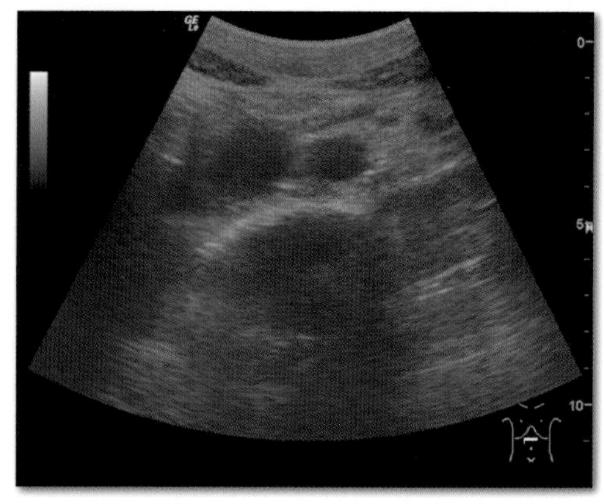

STEP 5

- For the last time, do again the previous steps and finish with step #5.
- With the probe's mark toward the patient's right, put the probe transversally in the epigastric fossa half way between the xiphoid appendix and the umbilic. The transducer is perpendicular to the bed and creates a right angle with the skin.
- If necessary, push softly but firmly to expel the digestive gases.
- Locate the aorta: optimize the image by setting the depth and gain; freeze the image, print it, paste it, and comment it.
- You will be brave enough to measure the aorta and the vena cava (anteroposterior diameter) and to make a longitudinal section.

Paste your picture here

- To finish, remove the gel from the patient's skin and from the probe that you also disinfect.

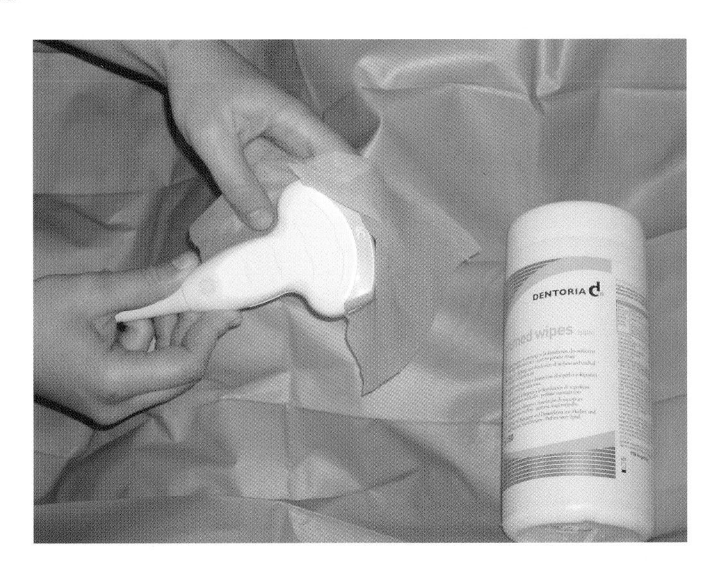

Learning test

Do again the five previous steps and, this moment, time yourself.

So, how long did you take?

You'll master the gesture when you can do the five pictures in less than 3 minutes. Buck up! You'll succeed.

Don't forget to clean the probe at the end of the examination and to redact the report.

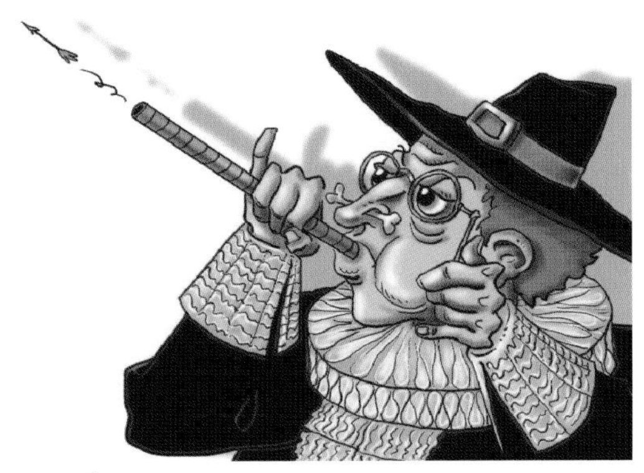

Have a nice trip to the land of ultrasounds.

FAST PROGRAM OF ECHOGRAPHY REPORT

Date: Patient's ID:

Operator: Dr

Echograph:

Examination indication:

Pleural effusion:	Yes	No	?	Side:
Perihepatic effusion:	Yes	No	?	
Perisplenic effusion:	Yes	No	?	
Perivesical effusion:	Yes	No	?	
Pericardial effusion:	Yes	No	?	

Abdominal Aorta diameter:

Inferior Vena Cava diameter:

Comments and Conclusions:

Signature:

Acknowledgements

*Thanks to Professor Raphaël Pitti, Professor Jean-Marie Bourgeois,
Doctor Jacques Kienlen, Doctor Jean Claude Deslandes, and all those who took a little bit of their time to show me the way.
Thanks to Doctor Michel Clairoux, Doctor Martine Pirlet and Doctor René Martin Professors at the University of Sherbrooke for their teaching and kindness.
Thanks to Doctor Eric Bouniol, Doctor Pierre Tur and Doctor Jean-François Adam who did so much for me.
Thanks to Doctor Luc Mercadal and the dream team.
Thanks to Mr Georges Bousquet for his sensible advice.
Thanks to Mrs Myriam Malvaut, Mr Dominique Torreilles and SAURAMPS MEDICAL.
Thanks to the whole SAR C team.
Thanks to the patients and their family who, in their misfortune, taught me so much.
Thanks to all my family and friends who supported me in this project.
Thanks to you who have taken the time to read these few pages.*

Lastly, I make a point of thanking the Springer-Verlag Publishing Company which agreed to publish the English version of this work, and especially Mrs Nathalie Huilleret and Mrs Sophie Guillemot for their kindness, their availability and their effectiveness.

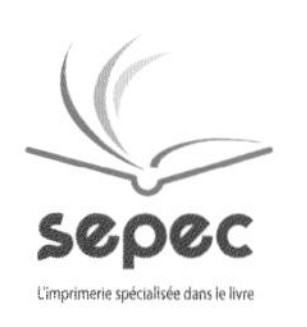

Achevé d'imprimer sur les presses de la SEPEC
Dépôt légal : Avril 2010

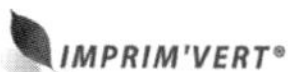